Praise for *Between*
of

Loved the book! You have had such incredible experiences! Enjoyed reading the numerous vignettes . . . they flow extremely well and of course have a teaching or learning point I believe in each. Should be mandatory reading for all health professionals!
You and Karen have done a fantastic job!
~Mark Lingenfelter, MD
Emeritus Professor, University of Wisconsin School of Medicine and Public Health, Madison, Wisconsin
Former Medical Director, Intensive Care Unit, Eastern Maine Medical Center, Bangor, Maine

You did a great job capturing the essence of nursing. I loved your use of humor and the comprehensive descriptions of the many relationships involved in the professional practice of nursing---patients, families, physicians, and coworkers, all so important, sensitive, and intimate.
Reading your book has brought back so many memories of my own experiences in critical care nursing and the wonderful feeling of being able to make a difference in the lives of others.
~Deborah Carey Johnson, RN
Former President and CEO, Eastern Maine Medical Center, Bangor, Maine

As the subtitle suggests, Karen and Ray have indeed created a treasury of care. But not just of critical care, but of the true essence of nursing. The vignettes provide realistic insight into the reality of nursing challenges and rewards. This book would be helpful to those considering a career in nursing, current nursing students, and seasoned nurses as well. Highly recommended!
~Suzanne Brunner, MS
Former Assistant Professor of Nursing, University of Maine, Orono, Maine

. . . [This] book . . . will serve not only as a great read for the general public, health professionals, and nurse educators, but will also hopefully find its way into classroom discussion for nursing students. Ray and Karen have created a book that could be read as a primer to understanding nursing concepts. It could assist students in identifying whether they would like to continue in the nursing curriculum or consider a different major . . . An ideal nursing curriculum would include an introduction to nursing concepts of care before going on to nursing clinical performance . . . These conceptual models would make for a great basis for clinical conferencing . . . It is with great pleasure that I endorse this book.

~Anne M. Hecker, MSN
Nursing Instructor, University of Rhode Island—College of Nursing, Warwick, Rhode Island

In words attributed to Mother Teresa, "A life not lived for others is a life not lived." Ray, during his lengthy career in critical care nursing, embodied that sentiment while continually maintaining a sense of mischief and humor with both patients and colleagues.
Karen and Ray have masterfully chronicled his years in the ICU in this touching collection of notable memories and lessons learned. Patients and colleagues alike have benefited from his caring approach to nursing, and I believe anyone with an interest in nursing, patient advocacy, or medicine in general will be enamored by their work. Highly recommended!

~Andrew C. Dixon, MD, FCCP
Pulmonary and Critical Care Medicine, St. Joseph's Hospital, Bangor, Maine

Thank you for the difference your presence has made in the lives of so many. The ripple effects are enormous, and the stories are passed down for generations because your life continues to make that difference even as they are told again and again.

~Jan Pettigrew, PhD, RN
Oncology and Grief Crisis Counseling, Little Rock, Arkansas

BETWEEN MIDNIGHT AND

DAWN

BETWEEN MIDNIGHT AND DAWN:

A Treasury of Critical Caring

Karen Buyno

and

Ray Peter Buyno,

BSN, RN, CCRN (retired)

Between Midnight and Dawn: A Treasury of Critical Caring

First Edition

Copyright © 2023 by Karen G. Buyno and Raymond P. Buyno

B & B  Books

All Rights Reserved.

Cover photo: Victorien Ameline/*Unsplash*
Cover design and editing: B & B Books
Authors' photos: courtesy of Samantha Mahar

Author's Note: The stories within are not intended to be literal accounts, though they are all based on true events, some details of which came from newspaper reports. Dialogue has been invented or recreated from memory; artistic license has been used in some cases to enhance the narrative. Unless otherwise requested, names and specific details of the caregivers and patients, with the exceptions of Daryl and Larry, are fiction based on fact, not to be taken as a portrayal of any living person.

Paperback ISBN-13: 9798854429818
Library of Congress Control Number: 2023914244

Dedication

To Mom Veronica, whose greeting cards and letters I always signed "from your favorite son," because that's how your presencing made me feel.

And to Dad George from your nurse; in your final, incapacitated days, if I needed anything, you made sure I knew you were there for me.

Table of Contents

Acknowledgements

We, the authors, would like to thank all the caregivers who authorized stories and/or ideas illustrating our intent, especially Anne, Ann-Marie, Dr. Robert Bach, Barbara, Brooke, Dr. Kevyn Comstock, Darla, Dean, Deanna, Debbie, Dick, Dr. Norman Dinerman, Dr. Andrew Dixon, Dora, Eileen, Julie, Karen, Karyn, Linda, Dr. Mark Lingenfelter, Lori, Lou, Marcy, Mary, Nikki, Pam, Peggy, Dr. Phil Peverada, Pret, Richard, Dr. Rodney Rozario, Ruth Ellen, and Sue. We would like to give special thanks to Daryl. Words alone are insufficient to communicate the power of what you have accomplished in life and your generosity in giving of yourselves and resources to help others, but it is our hope we can come close to inspiring others to reach for the same goals.

We are also indebted to Carole Brown, Debbie Carey Johnson, RN, Dr. Mark Lingenfelter, Dr. Andrew Dixon, Jackie Roberts, Suzanne Brunner, MS, Anne Hecker, MSN, Jan Pettigrew, PhD, RN, and Jennifer Laslie. You took the time to review our manuscript or parts of it, share your excellent advice, and/or write much-appreciated endorsements.

We reserve a special note of thanks for Jan Pettigrew, PhD, RN, without whom the book would not exist. You sowed the seeds of presencing at the beginning of Ray's career and have helped fertilize the concept's growth with your thoughtful analyses, dissertations, and advice. Others may have also described the concept, but you have ministered, and continue to minister, to others in crisis through your careful adherence to the principles of presencing. In so doing, you show us how to walk the talk.

1

Thanks would not be complete without adding family to the list of people to whom we are indebted. A heap of gratitude is due Raymond; aside from telling the stories, you sacrificed much of your time acting as what Stephen King called an *ideal reader*. Through your thoughtful evaluations of my writing, you have helped correct inconsistencies and have added humor where it was needed. Jason and Melissa, we are indebted to you for your invaluable literary and professional advice and encouragement in our journey. Samantha, you did the near impossible by capturing the rare serious side of Ray in film. Dora, you have been there since day one, encouraging us to follow our dreams. Many thanks to all.

We would not be fully who or what we are without the teachers who have guided us in our journeys. We would especially like to acknowledge the influence of the late G. Everett McCutcheon (of Stephen King fame) and the late Charlotte Littlefield.

As instrumental in helping this book become a reality were our friends, who believed in me as a writer, in Ray as a storyteller, and in the importance of caregivers and presencing. In fact, so overwhelming was support for this book prior to publishing that we were asked several times if there could be a second volume. To that end, we invite caregivers to send us their stories, and we will try to incorporate as many of them as possible into a second volume, one in which we can dig more deeply into the art of presencing. Thank you.

Care icon by Icons8

"Let us go then, you and I,
When the evening is spread out against the sky
Like a patient etherized upon a table."
~T.S. Eliot, *The Love Song of J. Alfred Prufrock*

Karen and Ray Peter Buyno

Preface

Messages spun from the threads of peoples' lives are much more powerful lessons than those delivered in sequential rhetoric, and the heart is much more efficient at remembering these than is the brain at recalling the latter. Simply put, stories are better teachers than doctrine.

When we first approached people about doing this book, the response was overwhelming from both caregivers and former patients. We received a lot of stories caregivers would enjoy sharing with each other because they were very humorous or poignant, even if they did not always illustrate the caregiver/patient relationship, and we incorporated some of them in the hope they would add to the reading enjoyment. We also applaud caregivers for finding enjoyment and fulfillment in their lives and for wanting to pass those aspirations along.

Here Karen feels she must apologize, at least to her mother and her children, for some of the graphic images and words used in this writing. In the words of Stephen King (*On Writing*), honesty has a lot to do with being "... brave. Map the enemy's position, come back, and tell us all you know." That's what we tried to do. In her defense, Ray took the photographs, and Karen merely developed the film. We hope we have not offended medical professionals by our efforts to simplify language for readers who may not be familiar with medical terms. We have also added some of our favorite quotes to help drive home and support the message of the vignette.

Additionally, we feel it necessary to include a note to the reader who is not a caregiver, who may view some of our comments or stories as unkind or unsympathetic toward the patient. Nothing could be further from the truth; indeed, a goal of writing this book is to promote the opposite. Caregivers in general have joined this profession because, at least in part, they have a desire to help others. They do not judge quirks or bad tempers. They love each soul they encounter as one of their own, and in sharing their stories they endeavor to teach others a little something about life. We're all in this human condition together, like it or not, and we'd best learn to laugh at ourselves in acceptance and love, recognizing a piece of ourselves in one another.

"Tell me a fact and I'll learn. Tell me a truth and I'll believe.
But tell me a story and it will live in my heart forever."
~Indian proverb

Introduction: To Be, or Not to Be . . . There

"There is no medicine like hope, no incentive so great, and no tonic so powerful as expectation of something better tomorrow." ˜Orison Swett Marden, author

Looking back over the past thirty-eight years as a nurse, I am struck with the certainty patient-focused initiatives were always around in some form, formally or not. It was always emphasized in the classroom that a nurse's number one responsibility was to the patient's every need, be it physical, emotional, spiritual or mental. After nursing school, there were countless examples made manifest to me through my daily work and the work of my coworkers of the nurse/patient relationship. It wasn't until my nurse peers worked their supportive magic on me, however, that I was truly aware of the power of such interactions.

In the spring of 1996, my marriage of twenty-one years fell apart. My friends were very supportive, but by Christmastime I was still dreading the season of giving. With three young children, I knew my feeling of isolation would be magnified by the lack of Christmas gifts with my name on them under the tree. It would feel horrible, I imagined, to awaken on Christmas morning and to know no one any longer loved me enough to give of herself to me.

Christmas Eve that year was one of the snowiest on record. Darkness descended before the sun went down due to the heavy snowfall, and the children and I began to make our preparations for

Christmas Eve dinner early. While the aromas of baked stuffed shrimp, sweet potatoes, and squash titillated their senses, the children waited in eager anticipation for the celebration to begin. They knew that Santa would be making his rounds and that they'd be wise to be in bed and asleep once dinner was over.

Before Drew, my youngest, finished his last bite of pecan pie, however, he looked up, certain he'd heard Santa on the front porch already. Calming him was useless. He ran to the door and flung it open. "Papa," he cried, "Santa *did* come! Look!"

"Wow," I said, "Look at all the gifts he brought you." I was floored by the sight. It is fair to say the porch was overflowing with brightly colored gifts of every size and shape. Beyond them were tracks quickly being filled in by the falling snow, and beyond them only darkness. I couldn't imagine just one person having enough strength to deposit so many gifts in such quick order.

"No, Papa, they're all for you!" In his enthusiasm he had jumped out onto the snow-laden porch in only his slippers and pajamas and had read all the tags.

My jaw dropped and tears welled up in my eyes, for I realized there were indeed people who loved me enough to think of me this way. It reminded me of one Christmas I'd spent as a boy with my eleven brothers and sisters. Instead of the usual one gift, we received two that year: a pair of socks and a small toy from my mother's two sisters. My father reminded us that our neighbor's family was poorer, and we were each told to rewrap one of our gifts for them.

To this day, no nurse has claimed responsibility for bringing the gifts---but I knew it had to be a nurse. It was a selfless act of love and caring that meant the world to me. It told me that people cared about me, there was hope things would be fine, and I would move from this darkest of midnights to the dawn of a new day. Twenty-seven years later, I am happy to say they were right.

It is this kind of emotional and mental support that transcends the physical needs of patients and is needed to give patients hope of better times to come. This support is necessary to ward off depression and hopelessness. Patients who give up are predisposed to not eating well, which of course can complicate the physical recovery. In the words of German philosopher Friedrich Nietzsche, "He who has a *why* to live [for] can bear [with] almost any *how*."[1] It is well documented from the accounts of prisoners held at Nazi concentration camps that prisoners did better if they had a goal and were able to maintain a positive outlook. Those who lost faith and hope were less inclined to care about trying to improve their circumstances in whatever small way they could. Similarly, patients who are isolated and cut off from support systems may feel like giving up.

As caregivers, perhaps our most important contribution is to provide appropriate emotional support through whatever means are available. My 96-year-old neighbor Fred helped to drive this point home to me when I stopped to talk to him on my way to work one morning. Wearing bilateral hearing aids with newly installed batteries, he pointed to them and said, "Speak quick. It's costing me money to listen to you." When he was not engaged in conversation, he would shut his hearing aids off to save on "battery juice." He asked me, in all the honesty that accompanies brevity, if after having worked so long in the nursing profession I was getting hardened to patients' circumstances. This had not occurred to me before, and I promised myself I would never become complacent or desensitized. It served as a gentle reminder that it didn't matter how many patients *I* had served before; each *patient* is a new experience.

Sometimes there is no basis for hope of better times to come; in those instances, the caregiver can offer comfort and a listening ear, can sometimes even facilitate an acceptance of the inevitable, and can help the patient attend to last wishes. During such times, the caregiver can also help family members begin their grief process, a progression, which though uncomfortable, is necessary in overcoming the darkness of despair. Though cure may not always be possible, healing of both patient and family is. Gifted caregivers can be invited by the suffering to effect "good deaths"---and not those of the Kevorkian genre.

In every circumstance, caregivers must be in tune to the needs requiring their attention, and learning to recognize what is needed is a focus of this book. Using true stories of nurse-patient interactions, I will try to demonstrate what is required of the caregiver in order to rise above the mundane duties of nurse, clergy, social worker, doctor, or other medical team member and achieve the level of educator, encourager, and escort; and I will illustrate how different my own practice was before my aspirations were realized. Required are skills that separate the caregiver from the medical practitioner, the healer from the drug dispenser, the friend from the acquaintance, the servant from the slave. The process of dedication requires listening not only to words but also to body language, insight that comes with knowledge of the patient's life and circumstances, empathy that springs from an understanding heart, and a patience that mirrors ourselves in every face we encounter.

Patricia Benner developed the concept for modern nursing in 1984 and termed such a level of involvement *presencing*.[2] More than a hundred years prior, Florence Nightingale, who provided her healing presence to soldiers in military hospitals during the Crimean War, demonstrated what it means to enter the suffering of the other person and to be *really there*. Not only did she tend to the soldiers' wounds, but she also held their hands and sent letters home to their loved ones on their behalf.

Jan Pettigrew, PhD, RN defines *presencing* as "risking entering the suffering of the other person with the whole of one's being, to be *really there* [emphasis added] as opposed to seeming to be."[3] Pettigrew laments that we as a society interact so often with machines such as cell phones,

10

video games and computers that we are losing the human touch in nursing. We are losing the art of nursing. We are losing what it truly means to be a nurse. We forget that true nursing is not just a job but a ministry.[4]

Caregiving without love and the recognition of the sanctity of each life is not ministry. In a poignant interview with Mother Teresa in Calcutta, BBC Journalist Malcolm Muggeridge recalls the tender and exultant words Mother Teresa spoke when ministering to a baby of miraculously small size: "See! There's life in her!"[5] Her words defy anyone to ask why we shouldn't try to save one life in millions so seemingly doomed.

According to Pettigrew, whose extensive research adds to that of Gabriel Marcel, Josephine Paterson, and Loretta Zderad, presencing can be characterized by five distinguishing features:

> Presence or presencing implies self-giving to the other person in the moment at hand. Presence means being available and at the disposal of the other person with all of self for that period of time. Presencing also involves listening with a tangible awareness of the privilege one has in being allowed to participate in such an experience. Further, it means listening in a way that involves giving of one's self. Finally, presence is identified as being there in a way that the other person defines as meaningful.

She identifies the critical components of presencing as vulnerability, silence, invitation, and privilege.[6]

Pettigrew adds that Benner defines an *expert nurse* as someone who has perception and insight into his or her patients. Such a nurse sees ahead three steps and is already planning measures to counteract negative effects triggered during the patient's or family's suffering. Paying

11

attention, reading between the lines, and addressing the little details that matter—the unspoken things---provide a recipe for success in interventions and invaluable modeling for medical students.[4] Sometimes we come to understand our patient only after gently peeling back layers of information and armor, somewhat like the process of peeling an onion. Other times, it is the patient who teaches the caregiver what is truly important. The information that is uncovered brings each of us closer to the heart of matters needing dialogue.

If you've ever lost yourself in a good book or movie, you know that identifying with a character can bring you to tears or to laughter as you immerse yourself in this character's life. Similarly, identifying with someone in your care need not be intimidating but may require a good dose of patience. Just as characters need to be well developed in a story, patients' backgrounds will help bring you closer to an understanding of the patients' circumstances. If two-way communication is possible, it can be very revealing. If it is not, communicating to patients about what is happening to them can be very reassuring. If a particularly horrific experience has landed a person in your care, take the time to tell him that you are aware of the horror he has been through and that he is *now* in a safe place, where everything will be done to help him.

Some of our chapters serve as teaching models. We discuss in detail what worked and why. Other chapters provide models for students to study and determine whether presencing made a difference or was lacking and *could have* made a difference. Because we are targeting students as well as challenging more seasoned caregivers in the art of presencing, we have decided to provide examples of the most basic levels and leave a more advanced and in-depth discussion of particularly complicated issues involving major competing ethical principles (beneficence, nonmaleficence, autonomy, and fidelity)[4] for a later volume.

Sōtō Zen monk Suzuki Roshi taught that one should pour oneself completely into any effort. One should not be a "smoky fire" but "like a good bonfire" burn completely.[7] Despite having twelve children, my mother Veronica made each of her children feel as though he or she was the most important one, a fact we didn't realize until all were grown and remarking on being her favorite. It didn't matter if there were three little ones yelling from another room, two clinging to her skirt, four entangled in a raucous wrestling match on the living room floor, and a baby crying for his milk. When I needed someone, I knew she would shut out everything else and attend to my needs. That is a gift that each of us in our various occupations can emulate: to be entirely focused on the person whom we are attending.

Shutting out other distractions may be difficult in our multitasking environment, but it is essential if we are to be wholly in the presence of these individuals who are entrusting their care, indeed their very lives, to us. We must be in the moment. In my own life, I have tried to remain true to the words of an elderly and wise African American woman I met while I was a Volunteers in Service to America (VISTA) volunteer in Hollins, Virginia:

> When I works, I works hard;
> When I sits, I sits loose;
> And when I sleeps, I go to sleep.

You know when you are "really there," in the presence of your patients, when you have immersed yourself in the depth of their pain, have tasted the bitterness of their reality, have lost yourself in their loneliness, and have come alongside them without becoming consumed to patiently continue their journey with them, anticipating their reactions and thus their needs. This is where the spirits of caregivers past and present unite and buoy us up in angelic form to meet sometimes

13

terrifying obstacles; this is the domain of caregiver *presence*, the realm of *critical caring*.

> To practice the science [emphasis added] of nursing requires a nurse who can perform a thorough and accurate physical assessment by inspecting, palpating, percussing and auscultating the patient's body. To ascend to the art [emphasis added] of nursing requires a nurse willing to perform a thorough and accurate assessment of the person, via inspection of the character, palpation of the mind, percussion of the heart, auscultation of the soul.
> ~Karen Bugaj, MSN, APRN-BC, RN-BC, CRNP

Prologue

Midnight was upon us, and with it descended a primeval desire to camouflage ourselves against whatever lay beyond the darkness. I pulled the curtains closed, leaned the framed photograph against the wall behind Ray's desk, and studied it for a moment before rejoining my husband and his sister Theresa on the couch. In the photo, Ray was smiling and seated (being that there were no other seats available) at his command commode in the charge nurse's office, his eyes as bright a blue as the scrubs he wore. Generously splashed around that smile were the autographs of his coworkers.

Sitting back down next to Ray, I lifted my glass of celebratory champagne. "So, what was it really like? Taking care of patients, I mean. Was it worth it? Did you learn anything in the last forty years you didn't already know about yourself?"

My husband looked at me with a twinkle in his eye, betraying the enormity that would constitute a response, and Theresa and I settled in for a wild ride . . .

Chapter 1: In the Beginning

"If you give me 5 minutes, I can give you something that took me 20 years to learn."
~Elijah Cummings, US congressman

Long before donning new scrubs as a nurse in a major medical center and taking the Hippocratic Oath to first "do no harm," an incident occurred that helped steer me in the direction of my career and transform me from naïve civilian to trusted, professional caregiver. I was living with my wife and child in an A-frame I helped build about twenty-five miles from the hospital, where I had just taken a job as a patient transporter. It was a quaint little house with original wooden beams in the ceiling and hard wood floors throughout. It also featured a very steep stairway to a second-level bedroom.

When June heralded the first spring in our new home, my brother Joie and his family of six children came to visit from Illinois, arriving one night while I was working the evening shift. Upon descending the stairway, Joie slipped and aggravated an old injury to his back. He was lying on the couch in my living room in a lot of pain when I arrived home late that night.

By the following morning, Joie was still miserable, and I convinced him to seek the advice of a neurosurgeon friend of mine. Joie is about an inch taller than I, and I enlisted the help of my wife to move him onto a piece of plywood left over from my carpentry exploits. After tying him to the board, we slid him into the bed of my old but reliable 1947 Dodge truck and closed the door to the cap of the bed. I gingerly drove the twenty-five miles to the doctor's office, trying my best to avoid the potholes for which Maine roads are famous in the springtime. It was a far cry from my present insistence patients be evaluated for proper Swan-Ganz (pulmonary artery) catheter placement prior to being released for ambulance transport, but, again, I was not trained in the finer art of patient care at this point. After parking the truck at the back of the doctor's place, I went in to see my friend.

"Where is the son of a beech?" he asked in his typical broken English, following me outside in his exquisitely tailored suit, not one strand of his salt-and-pepper hair out of place. He peered into the cab.

I walked to the back of the truck and opened the cap door, and Dr. B peered into the dark interior. Joie looked up from the backboard to which he was strapped and moaned. We were perhaps fifty feet from the door of the doctor's office.

"If he's that bad, just take him to the hospital, and we'll do a CT scan," Dr. B said. "No sense risking further injury and pain by moving him to my office."

The computerized tomography (CT) scan revealed enough damage that Dr. B admitted Joie to the hospital and performed a laminectomy and fusion of his vertebrae the same day. Postoperatively, I stayed with my brother and noticed Joie's nurse kept asking him if he had urinated yet. She explained that the atropine he'd been given to help dry his secretions during his surgery was also preventing him from voiding. When visiting hours ended at 8:00 pm, I picked up my jacket and prepared to say good night.

Joie's nurse stuck her head into his room at that moment, looked at Joie's empty urinal, and before retreating cheerfully announced, "If you don't pee by midnight, we'll have to put a Foley catheter in your bladder."

Joie looked at me in horror. He'd heard of catheters before and knew it meant inserting a tube through his urethra and into his bladder.

"Please don't let that happen, Ray. What can I do?"

I put down my jacket and walked to the bathroom, where I ran the water so that he could hear it, a trick I used for my young daughter before tucking her into bed each night. When the running water didn't produce the desired urge, I stepped into the storeroom a few doors down the hall and rummaged through the supplies until I found some spirits of peppermint, which I added to his urinal upon my return to his room. I wasn't sure what the medical staff used it for, but my grandmother always used it on her grandchildren before bedtime. Joie found himself still unable to urinate and begged me to help him. Being a twenty-something-year-old brother with a keen sense of loyalty, as well as a "medical professional" rookie with an IQ of a monkey, and rationalizing I was not on-duty but in civilian mode, I did what now seems to me the unthinkable: I peed in his urinal. With a sigh of relief, he set the now full urinal between his legs and bid me a grateful good night. I went home also feeling very relieved, confident Joie had avoided a "major" invasive procedure, and glad it wasn't an enema he had needed.

The next morning when I went in to visit Joie, the first thing I saw when I walked into his room was a Foley bag hanging on the side of his bed.

"How did this happen?" I asked in astonishment. "I left you with a lot of urine."

What I hadn't banked on was the perceptiveness and intelligence of a seasoned nurse, a professional who would not only follow up but also follow through. After I'd left, Joie fell asleep with the urinal between his legs. When he turned slightly, he spilled all the urine into his bed sheets. Aware of Joie's fear of the catheter and his inability to urinate due to the atropine, the nurse became suspicious when she saw the

18

unexpectedly pale drops left in the urinal. She didn't know exactly what Joie had placed in his urinal (a little ginger ale from his supper, perhaps?), but she knew it couldn't be his urine, which should have been a very concentrated, dark color.

"I laid in your urine for twenty minutes before the nurse could come in to change my sheets," Joie whined.

After that early experience in a hospital setting, I vowed under no circumstances would I ever again pee in anybody else's urinal, ever fill anybody else's bedpan, and especially ever again try to fool a nurse. But something else bothered me about the experience. Although the nurse was astute, her presence in the room was not reassuring to Joie. On the contrary, there was no direct eye contact, no touch, no one who would stop and address Joie's fears. Indeed, the nurse seemed to him rather to have morphed into another artificial limb of a healthcare system that seemed overwhelming and mechanical. He needed to be educated about what was happening in terms he could understand; he needed to be encouraged rather than frightened; and he needed to know he was not alone. The whole thing was more complicated than just trying to fix the root problem, on which I had also placed my focus. I gained a new respect for the profession of nursing, a respect which eventually called me to try on for myself the various hats of a truly challenging and rewarding career and to insert my very ordinary existence into a multitude of extraordinary situations.

"It's probably better to have him inside the tent pissing out than outside the tent pissing in."
~LBJ, 36th president of the USA

As part of graduation exercises for registered nurse (RN) school, an awards ceremony was being planned in the chapel of the Catholic hospital from which I had received my instruction. Thirty minutes prior to the ceremony, the director of the nursing program, Sister Laetitia, called me into her small office. I took a seat next to the door and glanced around the room while I waited for her to take her seat. It was not as lavishly furnished as I had anticipated for someone in such a position. There was no large oak desk, no color photographs of loved ones lining the walls. The austerity of the space---plain walls with crumbling white paint and an old, scarred, student-sized desk---was rivaled only by the dominance of the great crucifix, which hung behind her. On the desk was a ruler, and I was reminded of an incident in first grade, when Sister Roberta had slapped my hand for chewing gum.

"Ray, are you coming to the awards ceremony?"

"I wasn't planning on it."

"Why not?" she asked.

"Well, Sister," the rebel in me pressed, "there are two reasons. Number one is my classmates wanted a song by Bob Dylan, which is not going to be allowed. And number two is we were expected to buy a brand-new white uniform for the graduation exercises. It's like a wedding dress, Sister. I couldn't see buying one if I was going to wear it only one time."

It was only after venting my pent-up words that I was able to see the object of my rebellion in a clearer light. At eighty-five years and five feet two inches, she hardly cast the formidable presence I had anticipated. Maybe it was her long white habit, complete with the starched white wimple and bib, or the wooden rosary beads encircling her waist and terminating in a suspended crucifix, which had seemed so

20

threatening. No, they looked harmless enough too. A pair of old-fashioned, round wire-rim spectacles surrounded her tired eyes, and her hands lay delicately folded upon the top of her desk. I studied her face, which despite its softness was crisscrossed with a myriad of lines undoubtedly carved there by all the snot-nosed, self-serving greenhorns like me whom she'd helped mold into full-fledged, compassionate nurses. I was surprised to see tears welling up in Sister's eyes, and she removed a thin tissue from a generic box on her desk.

"I wish you'd reconsider," she said softly.

In the quiet recesses of my mind, a reassessment was already starting to emerge. I hadn't predicted my boycott would cause a little old nun to cry---a little old nun who'd after all been there in the beginning to hold our hands through the hesitations, doubts, and fears that had accompanied our decisions to become nurses. Hadn't she been there to take me from intravenous (IV) to indwelling catheters, from codeine to codes, from aspiration to applause? Hadn't she sacrificed a whole lot more in her entire lifetime than a song? Besides, I'd made my point, and I knew things weren't going to change overnight.

"Maybe I will," I simply said upon retreating, knowing I surely would and I'd better shake a leg.

I quickly shed my Levi's and pulled on the white uniform pants I'd used during training. I put my old white uniform top over the T-shirt I had on and ran out of the locker room and into the chapel. Slinking into the now mostly full pews, I took a seat near the back. My heart was pounding, not only because I'd just run in, but also because I was nervous I might be asked to get up in front of this crowd.

The evening went by quickly, as student after student rose and walked to the podium on stage to receive his or her award. Glancing at my program, I knew there was only one more award left to be handed out. *Phew,* I thought to myself. *Maybe I'll get out of this easy.*

21

The speaker looked out into the audience and around the formally decorated chapel. White balloons packed the ceiling overhead, while white crepe paper and satin ribbons adorned the aisles and speaker seats. Filling the air and mixing with the scent of the dozen white roses and baby's breath in a crystal vase beside the podium was the aroma of fresh carnation corsages. Mother Mary and Saint Joseph, in all their beneficence, smiled down upon the audience from a stained-glass window behind the stage.

"We have saved the most prestigious award for last," she began.

I was again relieved, remembering some of my less-than-genius moments, like the time I proudly challenged my nutrition instructor's grading of a test question by bringing in a box of raisin bran. The question was whether or not cereals contain a lot of iron, and my box explicitly stated the product had *reduced* iron. Though I found out later *reduced* means a "non-elemental *form* of iron that can be used by the body," my instructor did give me credit for trying.

"This award is for best academic performance. I'd like to call Nurse Carol to the podium."

A state of relief enveloped me, and I was finally able to relax and enjoy watching my friends and classmates bask in the fruits of their hard labor. Carol was a very smart nurse. Even though she hadn't studied as long and as hard as I had, she deserved the award. She had always been the first one out of the room during an exam, whereas I had always been the last.

I also thought Pam might have gotten this award. I first realized how smart she was when the eighteen-month program was just wrapping up and we were cleaning out our areas and preparing for the final exams . . .

. . . After removing six notebooks full of notes from my desk, I noticed Pam's pile of notebooks was considerably smaller. In fact, there was only one notebook in her hand.

"Pam," I asked, placing my hand on top of the notebook, "what's this?"

"These are my notes," she calmly said.

"Can I see them?" I asked in disbelief, concluding—or maybe hoping—she had left her other notebooks at home or knew shorthand.

She handed me the notebook. At the top of the first page was written "June 1977," the date of our first class. Three quarters of a page down was a tidbit of information I recognized as coming from our last class just a week prior. This was the first time I wondered if Pam might have a photographic memory, and . . .

. . . I was suddenly rocketed out of my daydreaming by a resumption of the speaker's voice.

"I'd also like to call Nurse Ray. These two students were tied for the highest grade-point average."

I was stunned. Nurse Carol was already graciously accepting her award, shaking the announcer's hand, and I floated past her in a fog as she happily took her seat. I felt as though I were watching myself from outside my body, and though my feet propelled me forward, they did not seem to touch the floor. As I stepped up onto the stage, my back to the audience, a peal of laughter started to grow behind me. Did they remember and appreciate the humor I had brought to the class? By the time I walked back past a smiling Sister Laetitia and sat back down, the laughter had risen to a roar, and I felt pretty well appreciated.

Preparing for bed that evening, I recalled how appreciated I had felt. I removed my T-shirt (a souvenir from a company whose services I once needed) and upon folding it noticed the design and bold writing on the back, which had surely shown through my white uniform top at the ceremony. It read, "Ray's Porta-Potty Service."

Entering into your patient's hell requires almost superhuman courage, strength and stamina. It would be difficult to imagine being able to achieve any vision of a deep level of patient involvement without the support of coworkers and mentors, the best parts of whom over the next several years I would weave into my own personhood. I would take their warmth, honesty, and compassion and make it my own, would mold them into my wholeness and beauty. Upon receiving the first Nurse of the Year Award granted at Eastern Maine Medical Center (EMMC) some years after my graduation, I gave credit to the human forces that surrounded and sustained me: coworkers to whom I could in confidence release the stopcock of emotions that were threatening to overflow; family and friends who cheered me on; people who believed in what I was doing when I was in doubt; partners who were with me every step of the way, no matter what; friends who cared enough to tell me perhaps what I didn't want to hear but what I needed to hear for my own good; and visionary guides like Sister Laetitia, who could see where the end of the road would take us, but who gave us our own space and time to process trivial matters.

> "We are not here merely to make a living. We are here to enrich the world."
> ~Woodrow Wilson, 28th president of the USA

Newly graduated nurses often come equipped with the desire to help but a lack of experience in administering all the necessary skills they have learned. The translation from classroom to actual practice in the trenches is not always seamless. As a rookie myself shortly after graduation, I shared care of a patient with Nurse Linda and was surprised one morning to find the patient with what looked from a distance like white spots all over his face. Approaching his bed, I reviewed the chart, looking for a history of fungal infections or allergies to medications, but there were none recorded. I knew it wasn't snow, frost or hail, since it was the middle of July. Could it be chickenpox, or had he traveled to some developing nation and been stung by a swarm of killer African bees? At the bedside now, I discovered the spots were actually about twenty-five little pieces of toilet paper plastered on his skin, a result of Linda's inexperience with shaving a man's face and her attempt at stopping the bleeding from where she'd accidentally nicked him.

Linda, Nurse Pam, and Nurse Beverly and I had all started our careers together. Eventually, I ended up on the evening shift from 3:00 to 11:00, and Pam, Linda, and Beverly worked nights from 11:00 to 7:00. When Pam relieved me one night, I told her my patient in room 140 was very sick and probably would not make it through her shift without getting into trouble. Those were the days when mouth-to-mouth was standard practice, and artificial manual breathing units, or *ambu* bags, had not yet come into everyday use in all rooms for patients who went into a deadly rhythm requiring cardio-pulmonary resuscitation.

"You were right," she said when we crossed paths again at 11:00 the next night. "He coded at 2:00 am, and I needed to do mouth-to-mouth on him."

"Gee, Pam," I said. "If I'd known, I would have given him better mouth care."

Pam forgave me, but it seems she often ended up on the wrong end of the stick. An *endotracheal tube* is a "breathing tube inserted into the distal trachea." Only once did Pam attempt by herself to move in his bed a three-hundred-pound patient fitted with such a tube. Department Head Sue heard Pam scream and went running into the room to find the patient on the floor in her lap---but Pam was still holding the tube secure.

Beverly, too, always seemed to have her patients' best interests in mind. George came in from the emergency room (ER) and hadn't eaten for almost ten hours. Beverly, who was working replacement on the evening shift, tried to call the admitting doctor to get orders and was still waiting to hear back. Meanwhile, the patient was threatening to leave against medical advice (AMA) because he was so hungry. Rather than see him suffer, she noticed on the dietary cart a tray of food refused by one of my patients, and she asked me if she could have it for her patient. He gobbled this up in short order and asked for more.

"Are there any desserts left over?" she asked us an hour later. "He seems to have an insatiable appetite."

"Beverly," I said. "I just got a call from the lab with a critical result. Seems your patient has a glucose of 800."

Since the normal range for glucose is 70-120 mg/dL, Beverly's eyes widened in a look of horror. It was a joke, of course, but it made enough of an impression in the immediate aftermath that she decided next time she'd just let her patient starve.

These experiences demonstrate our inexperience, but they pale in comparison to my very first day caring for a patient, which was while I was still in nursing school. While our initial failures to perform certain rudimentary tasks independently were embarrassing, I was dealing with a potentially more dangerous issue. And while the term *cockiness* has its roots in the male gender, those of the female persuasion are certainly not immune.

I was assigned to care for an elderly woman, who had been admitted to a Catholic hospital across town after suffering a mild heart attack. Preparing to enter Julia's room, I was filled with confidence that I had researched everything there was to know about myocardial infarction and had familiarized myself thoroughly with the woman's background.

Darkness greeted me when I opened the door and strutted into her room. The blinds were closed, and I could barely make out the tiny figure of a woman sitting up in bed. In the absence of light, I felt disoriented, and my confidence quickly waned, swallowed up by a Twilight-Zonish fear I was not cut out to be a nurse after all. *This is crazy*, I thought. *I should stick with carpentry.*

Gradually my eyes adjusted to the darkness, and I could make out a set of dentures soaking on the bedside table and a Bible in the woman's lap, illuminated by a small light near the bed. With her long hair drawn up into a bun on the top of her head, she reminded me of my grandmother, "Bába." (I was perhaps anticipating that, since she had reported she was Czechoslovakian in her demographics.) Remembering Czechoslovakian women like Bába never cut their hair—Bába's trailed two feet on the floor---I hoped I was not going to have to wash and comb Julia's.

"Good morning," I said cheerfully, trying to disguise my fear. "My name is Ray, and I'll be your nursing student for the day."

She said nothing but pointed toward a door on the same side of the room from which I had just come. Disoriented in the darkness, I thought she wanted me to leave.

Oh, no, I thought. *She doesn't want a man nurse.* Though I had worried about this before deciding to become a nurse, my mother gave me the confidence to continue. She told me she liked having nurses who were men because she felt confident in their strength to support her when she needed help walking and in their typical, no-nonsense honesty. Nearing the door to obediently leave, I noticed the other door beside it.

Maybe she wants something from the closet.

I opened the door and found the bathroom. *Of course,* my inner voice continued, the bounce returning to my step.

Returning to her bedside, my foot stepped on what felt like a power cord, and I kicked it farther under the bed. *This is a tripping hazard,* I thought, patting myself on the back for averting an accident. While I helped Julia out of bed, she began talking a mile a minute in Czechoslovakian. I had grown up in a Czechoslovakian household, and the words fell sweetly on my ears. But I remembered very little of the language. Every now and then I recognized the word *dobry* (pronounced do-bree), which means "good." I smiled, thinking she appreciated my talent at recognizing the bathroom. The faster she talked, the more urgent I thought was her need to get there.

While helping her up onto her feet, I noticed a downward pull, as if the floor were playing a game of tug and war with us. Nothing in my reading had prepared me for this. Her foot and hand seemed heavy, as if drawn to a magnet under the bed, and I pulled more forcefully to get her away. All the while she continued talking.

Finally, I said with a smile, "Dobry," hoping this would put us on the same team.

I dragged her into the bathroom as fast as I could manage, sensing by her still relentless talking that her need was urgent. After she finished on the toilet, I interrupted her rambling to interject some encouragement.

"Dobry," I said. "Dobry."

As we made our way back from the bathroom, I marveled at how fluent I now was in Czechoslovakian. *Think of all the possibilities. "Dobry" could be used in speaking with anyone, whether they're Portuguese, Japanese, or Indian. It's a universal word. I could use it to say "Dobry morning," or "Dobry night." If someone doesn't like the food, I could use it to ask, "Not dobry?"*

My musing thoughts were interrupted when we reached the bedside and she again started kicking and falling toward the floor.

This is odd, but she's not going to fall on my watch.

And I heroically scooped her up, placed her in the bed, and raised the bed rails. Whatever the force under the bed was, it now appeared to pull on her face and hands, which started reaching past the rails.

What the heck am I doing here? A lapse of confidence again began to color my thoughts. *I didn't sign up for this crap.* Not only was my first patient an eighty-five-year-old woman, but she couldn't speak one word of English. All the while, Julia never stopped talking. In Czechoslovakian.

Right about then my nursing instructor, Nurse Eva, walked in. I looked at her; I looked at the patient. Nurse Eva flipped on the light and opened the blinds. It was then I noticed on the floor sticking out from under the bed a small picture of Jesus. It was attached by two cords to another picture, and I recognized it immediately as a scapular. From my Catholic upbringing I knew scapulars are believed to allow a person into Heaven---if they are worn at the time of death---and realized she had been reaching for the floor (not the other way around—*Huh!*). I picked it up and placed it gently around her neck.

"Dobry," she said, settling back into her pillow and finally becoming silent.

Nurse Eva was not aware of all I had already accomplished that morning. I felt proud to have mastered a very difficult language and in so doing helped Julia in her time of need. She announced it was time to give Julia her meds.

This is where I will shine, I thought, feeling my confidence rise. I had watched Nurse Sandy and other senior nurses give intramuscular injections and had done all my reading. I knew all of this drug's side effects and could describe its pathway and target organ. I knew what to do to avoid hitting the bone and nerve. *Piece of cake. Piece of cake.*

Confidently, I filled the syringe with the medication and recapped the needle (which was acceptable back then). I knew the landmarks and put the index finger of my left hand on the iliac crest and my thumb on the greater trochanter. Proudly, I swabbed the "V" that fell within these landmarks, grasped the syringe and cap between my teeth, pulled the syringe out of the cap, and proceeded to give the injection. Glancing at my instructor for approval, I was surprised to see her mouth and eyes open wide in a look I had long associated with shock.

"Dobry?" I asked the instructor weakly. I would learn that uncapping a needle using your teeth is not at all good technique.

Despite getting off to a shaky start with Julia, I grew to like her and spent the following week as her nursing student. The first encounter had been a good lesson in humility, and it would be one of the last reminders I would need to make me realize that making of myself a virtuous hero or a suffering victim served only to hinder the higher purpose of my vocation. I realized I couldn't communicate effectively with a patient unless I was focused *entirely* on her. On our last day together, I waved goodbye in the fashion customarily used by Westerners, my hand up, palm side toward her, and fingers moving downward. She smiled and waved in the Czechoslovakian custom, her hand up, palm facing herself, and fingers moving downward, which meant, "Come back sometime."

"They don't care how much you know until they know how much you care."
~Theodore Roosevelt, 26th president of the USA

Chapter 2: Leveling the Playing Fields to Build Trust

"Humor is one of the best ingredients of survival."
~Aung San Suu Kyi, Burmese politician, diplomat, author, and 1991 Nobel Peace Prize laureate

Jasper was a Down Easter. Though the term is sometimes applied to a person from Maine, we Mainers more specifically apply it to a person who hails from the northeastern coastal region of the state, from communities like Calais, Machias, Eastport, and Addison. Down Easters have a reputation for being crusty and rugged enough to endure life on the cold, windy shore, and Jasper was a prime example. He was a worm digger by profession. It is as nasty a job as it sounds, requiring strength and endurance to plod thigh-high through gulping coastal mud. In his leathery face the lines of every squall and every broken rake could be traced. Though his shaggy hair and beard were still brown and there was a sparkle in his blue eyes, he showed every one of his fifty-two years in those creases.

Jasper's father had dug, and before him his grandfather. The family prize included blood worms, which resemble night crawlers except that they are capable of injecting venom in a painful bite, and the much longer sand worms, which can reach eighteen inches in length. Bent at a ninety-degree angle from the waist, a digger must comb away at the mud and hard clay, sometimes more than a foot for the deeper-burrowing sand worms. When the fishing was poor, one could still depend on the worms, which were sought after by recreational fishermen across the country and Europe and which had grown to be the fourth most valuable creature harvested from the Gulf of Maine. A strong-armed wormer could make close to a thousand dollars a week when the weather was cooperative, but this required him to recover close to 6,000 worms in the 17 hours per week available for digging. It was a lucrative, albeit backbreaking, business.

Jasper's son was digging with him in the flats when he'd suddenly fallen over, and he guessed the hard work had taken a toll on his father's heart. A brain tumor was totally unexpected. The best that could be done was a *subtotal* resection of the tumor, a fancy way of saying they couldn't get it all. The long-term prognosis was not good, but the surgery would buy him some more time.

"You should be out of here in a few weeks," I said to him a day after the subtotal resection.

"The only way I'm gettin' outta he'yuh is in a jar of formaldehyde," he joked.

Later, when Nurse Lisa announced she would be washing his hair, giving him a bath, and changing his johnny (hospital gown), he asked, "Why don't ya just covuh up m'riggin' 'n let the undertakuh do the rest?"

Perceptiveness is one of the tools in a caregiver's toolbox that assists in discovering what is really important to the patient or the patient's family. Oftentimes, the last thing a patient or family member says, perhaps whilst the person has his hand on the door knob and is going out of the door, is the thing at the forefront of his mind, and the caregiver would do well to jot down the comment and return to it at the next encounter. Likewise, the words, phrases, or ideas used most often by patients or family members disclose what is most important to them at that time.

Jasper's responses indicated that dying was very much on his mind, that he desired clarification of his condition, and that he was *inviting* Lisa to be there in that capacity for him. One of his consulting physicians, Dr. L, called Jasper a "joker and a smoker," which he often called many other Mainers who smoked three or more packs of cigarettes a day. He used this phrase in reference to the observation that when one jokes with someone in authority, it is often an attempt to put the other person on a level playing field with himself. Humor not only builds this kind of trust and often lifts spirits of patients, but it also adds enjoyment to our everyday lives in a field that is often otherwise very demanding and serious.

Shortly after the surgery, I asked Jasper about his profession.

"I sold worms to fishermen. You cud say I was a mastuh baituh," he chuckled.

I cringed. "What do you do in the colder seasons?"

"Well, in the fall I clam," he responded.

"And what about the winter?"

"In the winter I'm a clammuh with a hammuh."

"What?"

"Everyone in Washington County who's got a pickup truck is a carpantuh," he explained.

"Oh, Jasper," I teased. "You're lying through your teeth."

Jasper grinned widely, and the absence of teeth in his smile took me by surprise.

"Gee, I'm sorry. I didn't realize you don't have any teeth."

He pulled back his lips with his fingers and said, "I *do* have one tooth, way back he'yuh!"

Together we laughed and slapped our knees in delight. The disclosure and humor had put us on equal footing with each other, and we felt a little closer. I knew he trusted me, and he was sure now I would tell him whatever he needed to know about his prognosis. I often found myself hurrying through lunch to be able to spend more time talking with him.

Like many of his friends, Jasper carried in his shirt pocket a small black leather pouch. I saw the pouch among his belongings and asked him whether this was his Bible.

"It's my tobacco," he said. He then unzipped the pouch, slid a fine line of the brown weed into a small white square of paper, and deftly rolled a cigarette. Putting it up to his nostrils, Jasper closed his eyes and inhaled deeply. The crisp white bed linens lay in sharp contrast against his skin, darkly tanned to a line on his upper arms where the sleeves of his T-shirt had ended.

"Sure wish I cud have one," he said. "My great granny taught me this art. She did okay till she got thrown outta the pharmacy." Jasper scooped out a wad of the tobacco, popped it into his mouth, and closed his eyes in apparent ecstasy while he chewed.

"What happened?" I asked.

"There was one year we was fogged in almost every day. She started cuttin' off the ends of our condoms and usin' them to covuh her cigarettes, so she could smoke in the rain and the mist. She'd just roll the rubber back as the cigarette burned."

"That's pretty innovative," I observed.

"A'yuh. Well, when she'd used up our condoms, she went to the pharmacy and asked for a new box. The pharmacist knew Great Granny must'a been in her eighties, but he politely asked her what brand she preferred. She told him she didn't much care, as long as they'd fit a Camel."

When I stopped laughing, Jasper took a more serious tone.

"See," he began. "My dealer sells some of my worms to a university so the students can study their insides. He told me they do this experiment where they put one worm in a jar of alcohol, one worm in a jar of cigarette smoke, one worm in a jar of sperm, and one worm in a jar

34

of mud. After one day in these jars, the three worms in the alcohol, cigarette smoke, and sperm was dead, but the one in the mud was alive."

"That makes sense," I said.

"Well, the way I see it," Jasper continued, "As long as ya drink, smoke, and have sex, ya won't have worms!"

Jasper spit his chewed tobacco, which had deliquesced into a lovely brown liquid, into his urinal and smiled. Nurse Eileen came into the room to check on Jasper, picked up the urinal and left in alarm, believing her patient was now passing brown urine. I winked at Jasper and headed out to talk to Eileen.

It takes courage to crack a joke with someone you don't know. In doing so, a person bares his soul, exposing his less than perfect thoughts, risking that the hearer will accept more than his superficial politeness. The joker cannot predict how the other will react, whether that person will appreciate his sense of humor or throw him under the bus. Taking such a risk can be seen as an invitation to join him in a more intimate relationship. The joker is making himself vulnerable and asking you to be available. In effect, joking is a grownup's way of asking if you would like to come out and play.

"Laughter is the closest distance between two people."
~Victor Borge, comedian

Being a Down Easter, of course, does not automatically mean you have a good sense of humor. We all react to our circumstances differently, and one should not assume a bias toward people based on where they live. Estelle, for example, was also a Down Easter. She had lived in South Addison all of her sixty-seven years, in fact, and was known in the area as

35

a recluse. A clam shucker on the graveyard shift by trade, she lived alone in a white cape overlooking Eastern Harbor. People would sometimes catch a glimpse of her out mowing her lawn. Otherwise, she kept to herself.

If you've ever tried to shuck a clam, you know it's not as easy as it might look in an expert's hands. Not only does the shell of the clam need to be pried open with as little damage to the shell as possible, but the slippery clam body must then also be scooped out from its hold inside the shell. Shuckers' salaries are generally based on the numbers of clams shucked rather than on time worked, and quickness is a definite advantage.

When Estelle arrived in the intensive care unit (ICU), she was unconscious. Two weeks later, upon regaining consciousness, I asked her if she knew where she was.

"I'm in a f***ing bobcat's nest!" was her quick and sharp reply.

Though I was taken aback, I gave no clue of my surprise but immediately set to work to meet the challenge placed before me. I knew I needed to somehow get onto her playing field if there was any chance of a successful, trusting relationship. I had to find a way to be present in a manner that was meaningful to *her*. One thing I always did before taking on new patients was to take the time to learn about them, who they were and what they were all about. How many children did they have? What did they do for work? These were essential pieces of the puzzle.

"That's better than a clam in a shucker's hold," I countered and *drew the curtain around us.* And that's all it took. I was hers, and no other nurse even had a chance. In one fell swoop I had conquered her fear that no one would understand what she needed: a sense of control, space to herself, and a take-charge interpreter who spoke her language.

Given the extra time that seems to be required, some readers may be skeptical about the ability of caregivers to presence, especially in today's world of computerized charting and financial constraints. I would counter that while technology improves and artificial intelligence begins to reinvent how physical assessments are made, there will *never* be a substitute for human touch and compassion. The provider who recognizes and promotes such compassionate care will have a competitive edge. Progressive healthcare instructors have already recognized this and are paving the way for its inclusion.

Until such technological improvements are made, and considering the potential impact presencing can have on a patient's health, the caregiver is encouraged whenever possible to redirect the focus away from ancillary tasks by improving efficiency without sacrificing care of patients or self. This doesn't mean multitasking (shown to result in poorer performance and more frequent errors than with focused activity), nor does it mean sacrificing restorative times likes work breaks. Creativity is key in finding such time. When doing our yearly quality control and competency in-service training, for example, we found it time-saving---yet still instructive---to sit down as a group at several computers and discuss the questions. Not only did this simple merging of minds save hours that could then be redirected toward our patients, but everyone also got one hundred percent on their competency exams.

In the words of Jan Pettigrew, ". . . presencing can occur in passing in a hallway or on a stairwell, through a glance or a brief hug. The emphasis is not on time but, instead, is focused on really being there when you are there."[6] She cites the example of two friends who hadn't seen one another for many years. As a surprise, one had come in her wheelchair to listen to a presentation the other was giving. When the presenter saw her friend sitting in the audience, she left the stage, knelt at her friend's feet, and held her in a warm embrace before continuing with the presentation. This simple act took but a few minutes but spoke volumes.[8]

"What you like to kid about shows who you really are and what you care about."
~Author Unknown

Then there was Elmer, a lobsterman from Eastport, with the wiles of a fox. From my early days on the Maine coast, I was well acquainted with the give-and-take of a lobsterman's life. At four o'clock each morning, these folk rise, untie their skiffs from the wharf, and row (or *motor* in the case of the younger, in-a-hurry generation) to their lobster boats, which are moored in the harbor. At the start of each season, they must load their traps onto the boats and deposit them at various locations, which they mark with buoys painted in distinctive colors and patterns to distinguish them from those of their neighbors. The rest of the season, lobstermen check their traps, pulling them up and unloading whatever has been trapped, then rebaiting them as needed. It's not uncommon for a lobsterman to maintain eight hundred traps. A lobsterman's ability to locate all of his traps, even in fog and other inclement weather, is part of the repertoire of skills essential to success and survival in such a game of cat and mouse.

Elmer had suffered a cerebral aneurysm and was recovering from its repair. Part of a nurse's responsibility when working with head-injured patients is to see if they are oriented as to time, place, and person. Initially, Elmer could not answer questions like "What day is it?" or "Where are you?" In time, however, he learned that if he was to go home, he needed to show improvement, and he devised ways to answer the questions.

When asked what day it was, he would hesitate and ask the nurse to first get him a glass of water or to adjust his pillow. It didn't take too long to figure out that he wanted the nurse to move out from in front of the calendar! When asked where he was, he also attempted to see the wall-mounted welcome sign, on which was printed in large letters the name of our hospital. This necessitated a change in our routine and the way we asked him these things.

"What kind of place is this?" I asked him one morning.

He looked around the room in a desperate search for the answer, studying the ceilings and windows, and spotted the columns that formed part of the walls of the ICU. "Cement," he answered confidently.

I smiled at him, and he knew he'd been had, snared like a lobster in a trap. But my smile communicated several other things to him: not knowing all the answers yet was okay; I understood his reason for the game, and it was noble; I was on his side; I wanted him to be able to go home too, but I also wanted him to go home in better health, and I was *not* going to compromise that aspect. I reminded him about his adopted daughter, who was counting on him to improve so that he could continue to look after her. With knowledge that I was on his side and a renewed sense of purpose in life, he redoubled his efforts with the therapists and quickly regained his freedom.

On the day he was to be discharged, Elmer confided in me he'd lost his wife years prior and was looking for a new woman to fill the void.

"What do you want in a woman," I asked, trying to encourage such a train of thought.

"A pulse," he said with a grin. "Better you should ask a woman what she can expect from a lobstuhman."

"What's that?" I asked, taking the bait.

"A smell."

"Ha, ha---very funny. But I've often wondered about something else."

39

"What's that?"

"I've seen lobster traps, and there's a hole where the lobsters crawl in for the bait. Why don't they just go back out the same way they go in?"

Elmer smiled, his eyes twinkling. "Well, Ray," he said. "There's no one like you to guide them back through the little challenge standing b'tween them and their freedom."

"Humor is the ability to refocus maddening and threatening situations and reduce their negative impact."
~Author Unknown

Julep was by all outward appearances a very chic woman. Her hair was neatly styled, her nails were perfectly manicured, and she dressed impeccably. Julep originally hailed from the bluegrasses of Kentucky, where she had helped her father raise quality racehorses. In fact, one of his racehorses had placed first in the Kentucky Derby some years back. In her later years, Julep felt she wanted to leave the hustle and bustle of this competitive, fast-paced life behind. She purchased a smaller farm with fewer horses and a few cows in Coburn Gore, Maine, where she worked part-time as a veterinarian's assistant. She still, however, took an independent path when tending to the needs of her own animals and purchased and administered their medications herself.

Being the ripe age of sixty-five, Julep began to show some wear and tear on her body and most recently suffered a knee injury. She remembered having treated horses in Kentucky and more recently all her larger animals at the farm with certain medications by mouth when they experienced sprains. Julep decided it would be safe to take the same animal pill for her injury. Unfortunately, the dose for a large animal is several times the appropriate dose for a human, and Julep ended up in our unit on a dialysis machine to try and clear the toxins from her body.

Julep was a very gregarious and humorous person, who fit right in with the rest of us in ICU. On my first morning with her, I walked into the room, introduced myself and asked, "What happened to you?"

"Guess you could say I was horsing around."

"Oh yeah? What spurred you on to do that?"

Julep laughed and told me that upon doing her initial physical assessment, her family physician in Coburn Gore had started at the head and worked his way down to the feet in his usual routine. He visually examined Julep's scalp; he looked with an otoscope in her ears; and he looked with an ophthalmoscope into her eyes. He then took a tongue blade, placed it on her tongue and told her to stick out her tongue and say, "Moo."

I let Julep's attending physician know about her sense of humor. After the doctor explained what had happened to her and that the dialysis would take about five days to clear the toxins out of her blood, he added, "We'll have you back in the saddle in no time."

After three days of dialysis, Julep was "stable" and chomping at the bit to go home.

In a room adjacent to Julep's was another dialysis patient, Michaela. She was a tall and extremely thin woman, with brown curly hair and a beautiful, toothy smile, and she had been admitted after drinking an unknown quantity of antifreeze. Antifreeze is a sweet liquid, which explains why dogs and cats may eagerly lick up a puddle of it that has leaked out onto a garage floor.

"What possessed you to drink this, Michaela?" I overheard the doctor ask her.

"I was a quart low," she replied, having picked up her cue from Julep.

"What do you do for work," I asked Michaela later that day, following up on the doctor's inquiry. I thought she might have worked in an auto repair shop. We'd seen a few cases of accidental poisoning occur when an empty soda bottle was refilled with antifreeze but not relabeled.

"I used to work at the bug house."

"You mean the mental health facility here in town?"

"Yeah. I discovered the people who worked there were crazier than the patients, so one day I just up and walked out. Later, I did a little experimenting with LSD and called a friend. I told him I wanted to kill myself and was going to jump out my window."

"What happened?" I asked.

"Not much. My friend reminded me that I lived in a basement apartment."

Uh huh, I said to myself, freshly aware of the need to keep a more watchful eye on my patient. In circumstances such as this, there is a fine line one must walk between adding a little humor and staying within boundaries to preserve the therapeutic relationship and not minimize a serious situation.

> "If I had no sense of humor, I would long ago have committed suicide."
> ~Mahatma Gandhi, Indian politician

"Humor is a rubber sword—it allows you to make a point without drawing blood."
~Mary Hirsch, author

Leveling the playing fields to build fairness and trust, while lowering the feeling of vulnerability, is essential to all human relationships, not just that of nurse and patient. When I was a VISTA volunteer, I thought it would be fun to reverse roles one day and become the chauffeur for my African American friend and fellow VISTA volunteer Lenny. Keep in mind the year was 1968, just seven years after the Freedom Riders were attacked and brutally assaulted for daring to make inroads into areas considered "for Whites only." And we were in Roanoke, Virginia, *south* of the Mason-Dixon Line. One day, I donned the lay-me-out suit Lenny typically wore and drove him to where he needed to go. I opened the car door for him and tipped my top hat with the end of my cane when he stepped out onto the curb. For a couple of hours, I chauffeured him to the bank to deposit a reimbursement check for $4.95, to the post office to buy some stamps, and to the dry cleaners. We got a lot of raised eyebrows---lucky it's all we got—but we also earned a new respect for each other.

Certainly, if one evens out the turf in order to build a trusting relationship with staff, except for some of the decisions that must be made and the necessary compensation for that responsibility, the unsightly line between manager and subordinate can be blurred. Humor is again often the best tool to accomplish this.

If you had asked me as a brand new, rookie nurse in the ICU about daring to use humor with someone having the power to hire and fire, I would've had a much different opinion. Back on my first day there, I saw on the department manager's desk something that made me believe that a person in such a position should be placed on a pedestal: a bottle. The kind of bottle someone having a bad day might hide in a drawer or in a file cabinet, might come back to for a swig during particularly stressful moments of a typical day in the ICU. I didn't know at the time that the intelligent, classy Nurse Debbie from Milo, Maine who had hired me would one day end up being the CEO of the very same medical center. But I did understand it must have taken someone with a lot of courage to manage the sixty-plus assertive, self-assured and intense nurses in our unit and to tackle the everyday stress there. I wonder to this day if, with her promotion to the president's desk and the management of thirty-six *hundred* employees, the bottle of Maalox went away . . . or if it got bigger.

We liked to think that Debbie's eventual successor, department Nurse Manager Z, was wrapped around our little fingers, but she would prove to be a very tough nut to crack. Management had given this responsibility to *her*, and she took it way too seriously—until, that is, we were able to orient her a little more appropriately.

After several weeks of trying to keep staff posted about "urgent" messages, such as the new interdepartmental directive, or IDD, that prohibited wearing facial piercings or that prohibited personal business during work time---as if any one of us had time for formal breaks between saving peoples' lives---Nurse Manager Z finally got a brilliant idea. She would tape the notices to the wall in front of the toilets in the staff's unisex bathrooms.

"Didn't you see the notice?" she asked me one day. After I replied I hadn't, I suggested she also post the notices on the wall *behind* the toilets to give us boys an equal chance at seeing them. Of course, an equal chance at seeing the notices didn't add up to much, since nurses who work busy twelve-hour shifts often develop twelve-hour bladders.

At the height of this phase, just after I was comfortably seated in the bathroom, the portable phone in my pocket rang. I looked at the caller ID and noticed the call had originated from the desk near the bathroom. I hauled up my pants, stuck my head out the door, and saw

Nurse Manager Z smiling back at me with the receiver in one hand and the other hand on her hip.

"What do you want? *What* do you want?"

Nurse Manager Z laughed, for the first time realizing the new and controversial portable phones might after all have some advantages. She thought nothing of calling us at home, in the very early morning before the sun appeared and awakened the rooster, and during our vacations. Now she had succeeded in penetrating our last fortress against availability, and we found ourselves robbed of the privilege to even take a crap in private. Was *nothing* sacred?

Something has to be done, or we'll never have any peace, I thought to myself.

"Nurse Sue D," I asked, "did you see the Indian doctor who was just in here? She has a bindi *and* a nose ring, but *that's* apparently not outlawed."

"Yes, I did. I'm so sad about having to part with *my* nose ring."

"Maybe you won't have to. Let's see what we can do."

I took out a red magic marker and drew a large red dot in the middle of her forehead just above the bridge of her nose.

"See if you get any flack about this today."

Sue laughed and went on with the daily business of caring for her patients. No one said a word to her about the fake bindi, not even Nurse Manager Z, and Sue was satisfied she'd been able to say *something*. Ultimately, we lost this battle, but the war was not over yet. The Indians were still restless.

Sometimes it's the unplanned events that make the biggest impact. I believe the following incidents contributed much to the eventual conversion, or should I say "surrender," of Nurse Manager Z.

I had the unfortunate experience of needing to undergo surgery to remove my gall bladder. Fortunately, minimally invasive endoscopic surgery was available, and I was left with only three very small incisions (with which I was most impressed). During the period immediately following the surgery, one of my drainage devices became loose and soiled my linens. The bed needed to be changed. When a nurse came into my room to change the linens, I jumped up and made my side of the bed. She was quite surprised. Later that evening, when my IV pump alarmed, I leaned over and fixed what was causing the alarm. I put the IV tubing back in and restarted the pump. (I was acting partly out of intuition, partly due to the influence of the anesthesia still coursing through my veins.) The same nurse was in the hallway with a med cart, witnessed all of this, and now surmised I was a medical professional. Still later the same evening, some of my nurse friends from ICU came up to visit me. They washed my hair and lifted my spirits.

"Do you want to see my incisions?" I asked them, still high from the Vicodin. Not waiting for a reply, I lifted the covers and pulled up my johnny (exposing more than my incision). I don't remember if they said anything, but they sure seemed impressed!

Back at work two weeks later, I anticipated the sutures would need to come out, and like most in our profession, I felt it unnecessary to bother a physician for this small matter. Nurse Rita agreed to remove them.

I took off my blue scrub jacket, spread a white sheet on the lunch-room table—our operating theater---lay down, and pulled up my blue scrub shirt. The ICU had instituted a program of collecting unused, discarded supplies to ship to Guatemala, a destination some of the medical professionals reached twice a year. Rita rifled through our Guatemala box for an open but unused suture removal kit. The incisions were in my abdomen and just below my umbilicus. Rita stood between the door and the table with her back to the door. Because of the relatively poor lighting and her poor eyesight, she leaned over close to my abdomen to see the stitches, when Nurse Manager Z walked in behind her.

"What the devil is going on here?" Nurse Manager Z blurted out.

Rita, still leaning over my abdomen, turned her head, looked Nurse Manager Z squarely in the eyes, and proclaimed, "I'm giving him a BJ!"

"Flustered" is not quite the right word to describe Nurse Manager Z's reaction. It was more like shock and disbelief. She threw up her arms and left, but not before I could get out, "We're on our break." After all, that IDD prohibiting personal business during work time was still taking up wall space in the bathroom.

Not long afterward, I talked Nurse Lori into trimming an ingrown toenail. It had become so painful that I would either have needed to go home "sick" (which I never did) or get it fixed. We positioned ourselves in the secretary's office, one chair in front of the other, like a pair of nested spoons, so that she could best see the toe. I removed my shoe and sock and rolled up one leg of my scrub pants. In walked Nurse Manager Z.

"Not again," she groaned, putting her hands on her hips.

"We're on our break," I declared. Nurse Manager Z exhaled deeply and walked out. I've heard that water-boarding, if kept up long enough, can be an effective (if not subtle) method of encouragement. Its effectiveness lies not only with the shock value but also with its relentlessness. I knew it wouldn't be long before Nurse Manager Z would see the wisdom of our ways.

"If I can get you to laugh with me, you like me better, which makes you more open to my ideas. And, if I can persuade you to laugh at a particular point that I make, by laughing at it you acknowledge it as true."
~John Cleese, actor and comedian

Having a good rapport with the hospital chaplain and communicating effectively with this person is crucial to one's ability to meet a patient's spiritual needs. But just as a nurse or doctor must be invited by the patient to witness his vulnerability and share in his brokenness, clergy would do well to remember that ministry of faiths is a privilege by invitation as well. One of our chaplains, Father V, an eighty-year-old Franciscan priest and a most pious and revered person in our community, discovered the hard way that one cannot barge into a place of woundedness without incurring collateral damage.

During a particularly busy afternoon, a patient came to the ICU and coded soon after admission. We worked on him for hours, giving him dopamine, a fluid bolus, two units of packed cells, and other resuscitative medications until he was stabilized.

"Why wasn't I called?" Father V asked.

"I'm sorry," I responded. "We were so busy trying to save his life that we didn't have time to call you."

"Ray, next time remember the most important thing is saving the person's soul."

This wasn't my first encounter with Father V. The week before, I was chastised because I hadn't notified him of another patient's imminent death. The patient's religion was listed as "no preference" in his demographics.

"Unless proven otherwise, the patient is mine," Father had asserted in his sweet way.

Like Father V, Doctor T was well known in the community as a very religious and devout man. Not only did he sing in his church choir, but he also directed the Christmas music program at a local Baptist church and served at local soup kitchens. On top of that, he was known as a joker with a good sense of humor, who played pranks on unsuspecting colleagues. He would sometimes lighten someone's shift by instituting an urgent page for a fellow physician to a telephone extension at the morgue.

On Christmas Eve of 1979, I noticed Dr. T paperclip something to the cover of our yellow and black telephone directory before making his rounds—something I'm sure was meant for his fellow physicians. When he left, I went over to the phonebook and read the note, a question he had carefully crafted in cursive on a piece of Christmas stationery: "What did Mr. Santa Claus give Mrs. Santa Claus for Christmas?" To find the answer, he directed the reader to go to the *H*s on page 173 of the directory, second column, and find the 17th entry.

Just as I found the answer, a call bell alerted me to a patient in Room 140, and I left to help my patient. When I stepped back into the nursing station several minutes later, I stopped sharply in the doorway, aware Father V was thumbing through the directory. Opening my mouth to alert him not to look at it, I saw his lips mouthing the numbers: "Fourteen, fifteen, sixteen . . ." He read the rest of the entry, closed the directory as silently and as gently as if it had been his Bible, turned, and went quietly, stone-faced, back to his business, painfully aware, it seemed, he might need to tread more carefully in the future.

Dr. T entered just in time to catch my chuckle and hear me announce that this time the joke was on *him.* "And I'm telling Father V who did this." After all, I didn't want Father V to think *I* had anything to do with it.

". . . Fourteen, fifteen, sixteen, seventeen: *Hiscock, Nathaniel.*"

Dr. T meant to invite only his fellow physicians to witness the sacrilegious joke in the phone book. Imagine Dr. T's embarrassment and shame, how vulnerable he felt, because his less-than-perfect side would now be exposed to someone who seemed perfect. If Father V could have shown some of his own humanness to the doctor and assured him of his own imperfections, it might have alleviated some of the doctor's discomfort. Our patients and their families are no different from Dr. T. They want to be seen first and foremost as people, not patients. And they need to know we caregivers are as vulnerable and human as they are before inviting us in to share in their brokenness.

Leveling the playing field sometimes requires a person's vulnerability be exposed to himself. Stripping away what is most dear to someone unlocks resources to which he was previously blind, and it forces him to place his trust in himself or a higher power. Sometimes, unexpected solutions to long-standing medical challenges are procured through the most unconventional channels.

Doug was a celebrated singer in a hard rock band which graced the stages of local radio and television programs in the late 1980s. Doug had lost his left eye, and his signature trademark was a black silk eyepatch. Like many talented musicians of his day, Doug also had a drinking problem.

After a particularly raucous gig at Sugarloaf Mountain one night, Doug's buddies carried him to his scroungy hotel room and propped him up against the outside door. Before leaving, they switched Doug's eyepatch from his left eye to his right. When Doug came out of his stupor hours later, he was shocked upon discovering he seemed to be totally blind.

"Lord," he prayed, getting onto his knees, "I am blind. I can't see. If you would give me back my eyesight, I will change my ways and turn into a very religious man."

My friend and former patient Dick happened to be walking by during this time of prayerful contrition, reached down, and gently moved the eyepatch back over his nonfunctioning eye. From that day forward, Doug stopped drinking and began attending church regularly.

We are indebted to Nursing Instructor, Anne Hecker, MSN, for the following case in which presencing made an undeniable difference.

As charge nurse in the busy pediatric ward of our hospital, I became aware of a disruptive atmosphere in the room of our newest admission, an eight-year-old girl who had been in an automobile crash. Looking at her chart, I noted orders for the placement of a nasogastric tube and a subsequent X-ray. The tension and negative energy upon entering the room were palpable. Across the primary nurse's tear-streaked face was the unmistakable look of someone who had lost control. She was shaking her head, her lips drawn in a thin line. The father of the girl stood in a corner of the room biting his nails, his face flushed a deep red. He did not look up when I entered the room. The child was crying hysterically and thrashing in her bed.

"It's all my fault, "the father said. "I should've seen the other car coming."

"Would you like some assistance?" I asked the primary nurse, who breathed deeply and nodded. Knowing that crisis can increase one's sense of vulnerability, isolation and fear, I sat down next to the girl. Looking confidently into the girl's eyes, I smiled and gently but firmly took her hand in mine. After a few minutes, the crying and thrashing subsided, and the cold dampness left her hand. I could see that she was tired.

"My name is Anne," I said, "and I'm going to find a way for you to feel better. Just close your eyes and think of your favorite place in the whole world, a place you would most like to be right now. Imagine you are there. Can you tell me where you are?"

"At the beach," she responded.

"Perfect. Keep thinking about the beach. Think about how it feels with your toes in the nice, warm sand. While you're there, we're going to be here running a few tests to help us know how to help you. The doctors need to have you drink something that doesn't taste very good. The nurse wants to help you by sliding this very small tube through your nose. It won't hurt, but you may feel a little scared and uncomfortable. Just think of your happy place, and I will stay with you until it's done. Close your eyes and go to your happy place, and I will be right here."

Before her nurse returned for the procedure, the young girl had relaxed to the point at which she was sleeping.

"Did you hypnotize her?" the girl's father asked.

"No, I just changed the energy in this room, so that she could understand what was going to happen and relax. I understand how you as the driver of the car must be feeling. None of us are perfect."

The feeding tube was placed by the primary nurse, and I returned to my charge duties with the satisfaction of knowing that the nurse, the child, the father and I could all feel a sense of relief.

The first step in bringing about successful presencing in this case was Anne's placing herself at the child's level. Anne didn't hover over the

little girl but sat at her side. Jan Pettigrew, PhD, RN, who has made it her
life's mission to presence with grief-stricken and terminally ill patients,
has researched and written extensively about concepts inherent in
presencing. Citing the work of Paterson and Zderad, she asserts that it is
through one's countenance that one can effectively convey thoughts and
feelings: ". . . the nurse's face is revealed directly and unmistakable in a
glance, a touch, a tone of voice."[6] Has your day ever been brightened by
the cheerful smile of a stranger? In the same way, through her gentle,
reassuring and composed smile, her touch, and her calm tone of voice,
Anne was able to convey her presence to the little girl and effect her
trust.

Anne did not neglect to offer a reflective statement to the girl's
father, who was also in need of assurance. With validation of his feelings
of guilt, he was able to then focus on the more immediate concerns of
his daughter.

Chapter 3: Communication

As we transitioned out of the classroom into the reality of the bedside, there was another skill in our toolbox of experience that needed honing and that my fellow caregivers helped me to polish. In all of mankind, there is no more powerful drug than our words. Once spoken, words can be forgiven; they can never be forgotten. They have the power to lift up and the power to destroy. We needed to quickly learn to taste our words before spitting them out.

While still in the process of mastering this skill, I learned Deanna, one of our *maids* (a term I prefer to *housekeepers*), was going to get remarried.

"Congratulations," I began.

"Thanks. My guy's a forest ranger. Guess where we're spending our honeymoon?"

I was happy to see Deanna was moving on. Being alone for the last several years since her first marriage had ended couldn't have been easy.

"We're actually staying on top of a fire tower. Pretty cool, huh?

"Yeah, pretty cool, Deanna. What'd you do, kill your first husband?" I asked in my usual, spontaneously light-hearted, carefree and unfiltered manner.

"No, Ray, he died in a car crash eight years ago."

This hit me with such surprise that the mouthful of coffee I had just taken came spewing back out. If it had not been for what Dr. Norman Dinerman coined a "sphincter-tightening" experience, I might also have wet my pants. I spun around to avoid spraying her in the face and doubled over in a fit of uncontrollable laughter. The irony of such a poor choice of words struck me as so funny that I was momentarily incapable of doing anything except what I did *not* want to do---laugh. Getting out a controlled apology was difficult.

"Oh . . . I'm so sorry . . . I thought you . . . divorced him." I turned my back to Deanna to prevent her from hearing or seeing me in such restrained stitches over her apparent tragedy.

By the time I walked up to the fifth floor ICU five minutes later, word had gotten out about my faux pas. The maids there laughed, shook their fingers at me, and put their hands over their mouths when I walked by.

"Is something wrong?" Dr. Frey asked as I turned into Room 502.

"Nothing I can't remedy," I answered, letting it go and focusing on my patient.

"You can discontinue our patient's tube feeding. He's well enough to eat on his own," Dr. Frey instructed.

I nodded at the University of Maine nursing student already at the bedside as Dr. Frey charted the change and left to attend to his next patient.

"Discontinue the tube feeding," I reiterated.

"What do you want me to do with it?" the nursing student asked.

"Just put it in the sink," I said, spotting a maid walking past the door. I smiled at the student and went into the hall to have a few words with the cleaning crew.

A few minutes later, having done the best I could do to undo the damage I'd inflicted, I returned to Room 502 and was startled to see the six-foot IV pole in the sink hanging precipitously over the counter and still attached to the pump and the tube-feeding bag, which were also crammed into the sink. I laughed, gave the student an A+ for creativity, and gave myself a D- for communication.

Deanna let me think about my blooper for another few weeks, when she confessed they'd been in the middle of a divorce when her first husband was killed.

"No man is an island,
Entire of itself."
~John Donne, poet

The lifeline that tethers each of us to the rest of the world is communication. Try to imagine what it would have been like for the patient in the following story if there had been no communication, if everything done to and for him were done in silence. We are indebted to Nurse Practitioner Peggy for sharing in her own words this poignant encounter, an excellent example of patient presencing, and for reminding us of this very essential and basic necessity.

"We're getting an admission, and you'll be taking him. He should be arriving within an hour. A motor vehicle crash from the Belfast area." The 3-11 shift had begun, as it did most days in our surgical intensive care unit, with patient assignments made by our charge nurse.

I prepared for the arrival of Tim, a twenty-something-year-old who lived an hour east of our medical center, and who had hit a bridge embankment with his car while driving to work that day. After stabilization at his local hospital, he was piled into an ambulance with emergency personnel for the long drive over narrow, bumpy Maine roads to our hospital.

Tim arrived shortly after report was given, bypassed the emergency department, and was brought right to our unit. He was intubated, unconscious, and bloody but had stable vital signs. The plan was to get him quickly to the operating room (OR) to address his severely fractured right leg. Quickly, I began my nursing assessment as I waited for the OR staff to come get him, and I told Tim exactly what was happening. As I worked, I told him where he was, how he got here, and that he was heading to the OR; I would be here when he got back.

Tim was taken for X-rays, a CT scan, and surgery and arrived back to me late in the shift. His leg was newly bandaged and suspended in traction, his eyes were closed, and the ventilator was breathing for him. I had time to check his vital signs, administer medications, and begin the process of cleaning up the caked, dried blood and numerous contusions he had suffered. I talked to Tim as I worked, and the shift quickly ended. I promised him I would see him the next day.

Tim spent the next couple of weeks with us, requiring further surgery and treatment, while each evening I was assigned to his care. It took several days before he was weaned off the ventilator and extubated, and although his injuries were serious and numerous, Tim continued to improve slowly. His age was his friend, and he withstood surgeries and treatments, fevers and nursing care with stable vital signs and slow improvement.

Each evening I spent with Tim, I talked to him. He never regained consciousness while with us, but his coma lightened during the weeks he spent in the ICU, and he was making purposeful movements. I talked to Tim about the crash---a terrible one he was lucky to survive---and I talked to Tim about life. He heard about how smitten I was with my boyfriend, now husband of twenty-six years; about the weather; about his treatment plan. I talked to Tim about my friends, my family, and my political views. I talked to him about anything and everything, and I kept up my running commentary to Tim with words of encouragement that he was improving and would be home soon. Though he never spoke to me, I always looked forward to caring for Tim, who became one of the special patients we as nurses always remember.

After a day off, I returned to work and found Tim gone from the ICU. He had improved and stabilized and now faced the difficult task of rehabilitation. Tim had transferred out to the rehabilitation floor to continue healing, and I received new assignments, moving on to the next patient in need.

Several weeks later, as the day shift report to our 3-11 team was just finishing, the door from the visitors' waiting room opened. Two women held the door, and a handsome young man with dark blond hair, in a wheel chair, right leg extended and elevated, wearing a wide grin, rolled himself into the ICU and maneuvered over to the two shifts of nursing staff. One of the women told us Tim was finally being discharged from the hospital to continue his recovery at home, and he wanted to meet the nursing staff who had cared for him when he was so ill.

Our large group of nurses began talking to Tim excitedly, all at once, and Tim grinned widely, looking at each of us. While we continued to talk, he suddenly turned his head, sought me out in the group of nurses and looked straight at me.

"You," he said. "You're the one." We all stopped talking and I asked what he meant.

"You're the voice I will always remember. You talked to me every day, and you promised me I'd get better. You never stopped talking to me. I knew your voice, but I wanted to see who you were and what you looked like."

And while we all stayed silent, Tim finally---finally---began talking to me.

"They forget your name, but they will never forget how you made them feel."
~Maya Angelou, MJ holst ARNP, MHS

58

Boasting a beautiful national park, Maine has seen some very wealthy people visit from around the globe. Occasionally, one of these visitors may run into a medical issue and end up in our facility. Such was the case one summer when the thirty-year-old wife of a physician from Utah suffered a stroke secondary to the rupture of a cerebral aneurysm.

After her surgery, Cindy needed to breathe deeply and cough to clear her lungs and prevent pneumonia. This was something to which we always paid close attention. As Doctor E phrased it to patients, "You better be coughin', or you'll be in a coffin!" Nurse Rosalie, unaware someone so young was hard of hearing, gave the routine instructions.

"Cough and take a nice big breath," she said.

"Thank you," Cindy responded. "I like my breasts too."

Rosalie smiled but, not wanting to start any unsavory rumors, quickly corrected what Cindy thought she had heard. A month later, she was also able to update Cindy about her husband's request to move her closer to home for the rest of her recovery. After a little more rehabilitation, Cindy would be ready to join him in Utah.

"Your doctor has given his preliminary blessings for you to fly next week, as long as you have a nurse accompany you. We've done a lot of hard work getting you ready and want to make sure you get home in one piece. Okay?"

"Okay. Is there a nurse here who would be willing to take me?"

"We have a list of nurses willing to travel with patients. We'll find someone suitable for you, if you like."

"That would be great, thanks."

Rosalie turned to leave and added, "It's the end of my shift."

"No, I don't need to take a shit," Cindy answered.

Rosalie smiled and continued on her way. It wasn't worth correcting. She dialed the number of Cindy's primary nurse, who knew the family well.

"Hi, Ray," she said when I answered. "Would you be interested in transporting a patient to Utah?"

Early in my nursing career, I volunteered to transport patients "anytime and anywhere." Not long after offering my services, I was awakened one morning at 2:00 am from a deep sleep and asked by the ER charge nurse if I would be interested in transporting a patient to England. Not fully awake, I hung up the phone. Ten minutes later and fully aware, I remembered the call and called the ER back.

"May I speak to the nurse in charge, please?" I asked.

"Speaking."

"This is Ray. I'm sorry I hung up on you. I'm very interested in taking your patient to England."

"Ray, what are you talking about? We didn't call you."

That call was a dream, but before the advent of medical helicopter services I would go on to complete probably fifty such transports. Cindy would be my third.

We left Bangor at 2:00 am in a limousine for a 7:00 am flight out of Logan Airport in Boston, where we had a two-hour delay before boarding our flight, due to a ruptured tire on the plane. Cindy's husband had decided flying home first class by commercial jet would be the best way to get her home because there was a bathroom nearby. She was on a diuretic, which made her urinate frequently. Of course, the Mrs. needed to use the bathroom while we were at the terminal. Having raised two daughters, I was accustomed to taking young girls into the men's bathroom during our excursions cross-country. But this was a grown woman, and I didn't feel that would be appropriate. Keeping a cool head, I looked around for a commode. There were none.

"I'm going to have to take this woman into the women's bathroom." I said the words out loud to myself, knowing it was the best option and hoping that saying the words aloud would diminish their punch. I began to regret cutting my long hair but then realized how embarrassing it would be to be arrested for impersonating a woman. While I continued to ponder how I might accomplish this, Cindy let me know I didn't have much time to think about it.

"Let's see," I began in a low voice.

"Okay, let's pee. But can I go first?" she stammered, and I realized I had forgotten to speak up.

Just as I was about to bite the bullet and head into the ladies' room, I noticed a maid going into the bathroom to clean it, and I asked her if she would kindly clear out all the people so that I could go into the bathroom with my patient. "Thank goodness," I whispered.

An hour later and sitting pretty in first class, I felt smug. Surely it would be smooth sailing from here on out. As we approached cruising altitude and the "buckle your seat belt" sign went out, Cindy announced she needed to use the bathroom again. A sign above the first-class lavatory read "out of order," and we were forced to go from the first seat in first class all the way to the back of the plane to that bathroom. Due to the stroke, Cindy walked as if she'd already filled her pants, and this required me to steady her steps by holding on to her belt from the back.

I sat her down and cleaned her up, after which she whispered, "I wonder what all those people think about us being in the bathroom together?"

"Yeah, it's okay. Just relax and take a nice big breath," I whispered back.

I didn't know at the time what Cindy heard me say, but there was a sudden loud slap, and my cheek felt as if it would migrate to my feet. I clarified what I'd said, and she quickly apologized.

Trying to act professional and to shield my face with Cindy's body, I stepped out of the lavatory with Cindy. People put down magazines and strained their necks to get a glimpse of the creep who had apparently assaulted this poor lady in the bathroom.

At 12:30 pm we arrived in Salt Lake City, and I delivered Cindy into the appreciative arms of her physician husband at their home. I returned to the airport and hopped onto my returning flight, but because the connecting flights were bumped due to the earlier delay, I didn't get to Newark until fairly late. By that time, the last flight to Bangor had already left, and I was stuck in New Jersey. The airline kindly put me up for the night in a nearby hotel. At 12:20 am, my wife called and told me someone had broken into my van, which was parked at the hospital, and had broken out all seven of the windows. By the time I got home later that day, a local glass company had replaced the windows, but a sputum container full of quarters that I always left in the car for my teenaged daughters was missing. Despite the hassles, it'd been a pretty good day. In addition to my day's wages, the physician had given me a thousand-dollar tip, more than enough compensation to cover the hundred-dollar deductible for my car windows, I thought, rubbing my cheek.

Blood gases are drawn to help determine whether patients need intubation and ventilation. A blood gas was drawn on a fifty-eight-year-old man in our unit. His carbon dioxide (CO_2) level was quite high, and his pH was quite low, indicating the need for immediate intubation.

I called the blood gas results to the doctor, who was at home, and he was in agreement about the patient needing a breathing tube. After documenting the order, I turned to Nurse Sharon, the patient's caregiver.

"Dr. M wants Bruce intubated. His gases are abnormal."

"Bruce actually is adamant about *not* wanting to be intubated. He just wants to be let go." Nurse Sharon was our resident patient advocate. If anyone could convince a physician to go with the patient's wishes, it was she.

I was soon back on the phone and related the patient's wishes to Dr. M.

"I don't care," Dr. M began. "Intubate him anyway."

Nurse Sharon stared at me with a pair of red-hot daggers. She said nothing but went about the business of following the doctor's order.

Forty-eight hours later, the tube was removed from Bruce's trachea, and he was able to breathe on his own. I went to his room shortly thereafter to explain to him how he came to be intubated.

"I realize intubation was against your wishes and you just wanted to be allowed to die," I began.

"I don't remember saying anything like that!" Bruce exclaimed in horror.

This incident taught me a good lesson about blood gases and their effects on the mind; its example underlines the fact that the body can affect the mind, just as the mind can sometimes affect the body. A high CO_2 level in one's blood can make a person very confused. It also reminded me about the knife edge we constantly walk when navigating ethical dilemmas. For some reason I sided with the doctor in this case, but I usually side with the nurse. If we'd gone with the patient's *apparent* wishes, we would have done gross disservice to this patient. Before advocating for patient rights, the healthcare provider would do well to remember that ethical decisions of this magnitude should be authenticated over a period of time and in a state of being that assures mental competency.

For some reason, the period between Thanksgiving and Christmas marked a time when the units caring for critically ill patients usually saw a drop in their censuses. This year, however, was a bit unusual. With snowfall totals at a historical low, the number of heart attacks precipitated by shoveling was down, and there were empty beds in our coronary care unit (CCU). But the ICU was filled to capacity, and the ER had just called to request yet another bed for a new trauma patient.

Since the responsibility fell on me to find a bed, I approached the charge nurse of CCU, Nurse Nikki. When Nikki wasn't caring for patients, she was taking care of horses. During her time off, she was a constant figure in the stables and was known in close circles as "Maine's horse whisperer." Like the subject of the popular novel and movie, she possessed a remarkable gift for understanding and calming a horse when it was startled by the sudden appearance of a snake or the unfamiliarity of a saddle. Her techniques included working in sympathy with the horse in order to obtain cooperation, gentleness, the use of reassurance rather than punishment, and the utilization of human body language to communicate effectively. These were the same skill sets she brought to her professional life and which made her so effective as a nurse.

"Any chance you could take one of our patients?" I asked her. "We're bursting at the seams and have to find another bed."

Nurses develop their skills through experience in their specialties. CCU nurses did not have the skills needed to care for neurological patients, complex surgical patients, or complex obstetrics patients; likewise, ICU nurses lacked the necessary skills to care for open-heart surgical patients and cardiac patients in general. As it happened, most of the patients in the ICU that day were comatose, ventilated, or complex neurological patients, which left only a handful of patients who could be transferred to CCU.

I watched, her nonverbal betraying a mixture of concern and ambivalence. "Come on down and go shopping," I invited her, undaunted.

Sighing, Nikki closed the drawer to the file cabinet in which I had found her alphabetizing her folders in the spare time the lull afforded her. When she reached the ICU, I handed her a Kardex containing each patient's information.

"Pick one," I offered.

"How 'bout this one?" she asked, handing the Kardex back with her thumb marking the entry of her choice.

"That'd be fine," I said, glancing at her choice.

"What's the status?"

"The patient has expired, but the family has requested we not move him just yet," I answered, walking her to Room 148, where the man lay in the dark, his hands folded neatly on top of a sheet, ready for family members who had yet to say their goodbyes.

"The doctor has notified the patient's wife, who asked about family members who lived three hours away coming to see him. We're expecting them to arrive this afternoon."

It seemed like the perfect choice for Nikki. The CCU nurses could take the time to pay attention to the finer details, like pushing the cuticles back on the deceased patient's fingernails. The ICU nurses, on the other hand, were attending to patients who had no fingers.

When I was ten, my grandmother fell and broke her hip and ended up in the hospital with pneumonia. I called the hospital to inquire about her condition, and the nurse told me she had expired. I didn't know what that meant, and neither did my brother. We called back to get clarification and, upon asking where she was, were told she had been moved to Urbas Funeral Home. Then, we knew.

The physician who had been attending the patient whom Nikki took to CCU had told the patient's wife her husband had expired. Little did the doctor or I know she was Franco-American, spoke limited English, and was unfamiliar with the term used in this way. Thinking that perhaps the papers allowing him to stay in the hospital had expired, she sent family members, who were unaware their precious relative was dead, to visit and sign the papers allowing him to stay.

Because she felt this patient would be very easy, Nikki had assumed the responsibility of care herself rather than burden her staff with the responsibility. But the family's confusion and shock following the discovery of their loved one's death turned out to be a fiasco, consuming much of her time and talents, and pushing the limits of her extraordinary ability to calm creatures out of control. Nikki counts this day among one of her finest as a charge nurse, a day she learned *death* and *dead* were not swear words. A day she also learned never to assume responsibility of a patient from me, no matter how compliant the patient appeared to be.

"Words are the source of misunderstandings."
~Antoine De Saint-Exupéry, *The Little Prince*

In an emergency situation, such as a code, coworkers often commented about how calm I was. "Stay calm," I'd say. "We have three minutes." I wasn't being cocky as much as I was trying to keep my head about me and those around me. I never forgot when one of my colleagues ran so fast to a code that she crashed our code cart, necessitating someone to go and find another cart, which ultimately lost more time than if we'd acted less frantically.

Nurse Pret showed me how to take my calmness even one step higher and give validation to those who need to be present at such high-stakes events. He recognized that each member of the code team was there for a legitimate reason.

When the lab person came to draw blood, Pret would announce, "Make room for the lab person. She is the most important person in the room right now."

When the X-ray technician wheeled his cart through the door, Pret's voice could again be heard. "Make way for the X-ray tech. He is the most important person in the room now."

The first time I experienced a code with Nurse Pret in attendance, we, along with two other nurses, a doctor, a respiratory therapist, and a chaplain, were coding a teenager in the pediatric intensive care unit (PICU). Pret invited the mother of the teenager to stand at the head of the bed, telling her she was the most important person in the room.

We are grateful to Nursing Instructor Anne Hecker, MSN for the following encounter. When urgency demands action, a balance must be struck between remaining calm and communicating effectively. Otherwise, support team members may not understand the appropriate level of response required.

Giving senior level students complex patients was my way of challenging the top achievers. Students Abby and Luke followed me into Room 502, where a toddler was happily playing in his highchair. On a ventilator since birth, the child was currently recovering from a respiratory infection and had a tracheotomy.

As we were preparing to leave, the child began banging his toy wooden hammer on the tray of the highchair, and it soon connected with a part of the ventilator tubing, causing the tube to crack. It was an opportune time for instruction. The patient was unable to maintain his oxygen saturation, and I instructed Luke to carefully disconnect the tubing, after which I demonstrated to him and Abby how to use the ambu bag.

"Luke, please call respiratory therapy for new tubing," I instructed, pointing to the phone in the hall just outside the room.

Upon his return to the bedside, Luke continued to assist respirations with the ambu bag. All of the child's vital signs returned to what they were before the tubing broke.

Forty minutes passed before a respiratory therapist arrived with new tubing. "Oh, my," the therapist said, "I am so sorry! Luke was so calm when he called me that I had no idea it was an emergency. So, I decided to deliver the tubing at the patient's next scheduled assessment and treatment instead of rushing over."

What I had hoped would be a challenge for my students turned into a learning experience for all of us. The team work was amazing, and I emerged with a lesson learned: encourage students to remain calm in a potentially threatening situation, but when communicating with other members of the team, state the situation clearly enough for others to take appropriate action. This is one situation in which an increased anxiety level may have been a plus.

Chapter 4: Cleaning Up the Messes

One of the unpleasant responsibilities many people associate with nursing and caregiving in general is that of cleaning up patients unable to care for themselves. A caregiver may need to help blow a patient's nose, clean up a wound, suction out saliva, empty a urinal, or clean up stool. Probably the tasks I personally found most objectionable were aiding in stool transplants or in the introduction of artificial saliva. For those wishing to overcome such obstacles, I suggest immersing oneself as much as possible. Standing on shore dreading the cold of water does nothing to overcome that obstacle; there's nothing like jumping right in to circumvent such fear. After the first few times of doing each task, the undertaking begins to lose its potency. No career is without its unpleasantries, and the rewards of caregiving more than compensate for the little time spent on such "messes."

Miss Juanita, as she preferred to be called, was a small woman of African American descent. She lived in the Roxbury district outside of Boston. Nurse Peggy cared for her at Boston City Hospital.

"What happened to you?" she asked Miss Juanita.

Miss Juanita was a single mom who had fallen on hard times. Boston can be a very unforgiving place to live. By day she worked as a store clerk, and evenings as a waitress. In this way she was able to provide fairly well for her three children. They were clean and neat, though they never saw much in the way of anything fancy.

In February, when it got colder, money became an issue, and she found it necessary to cut back on something. She could not afford to heat her entire apartment but found that if they all huddled together on cots in the kitchen, the gas range and burners provided enough heat.

"My youngest left his homework on the counter near the stove," she began. "A draft must'a sent it onto the burners durin' the night." She wiped a tear from her cheek, then continued. "Anyway, all the kids got out okay. I wasn't so lucky."

Miss Juanita suffered second-degree burns over forty percent of her body. Second-degree burns are more painful than first-degree burns (such as sunburns), in which only the topmost layer of skin is burned. Second-degree burns expose the nerves and are more painful than third-degree burns, in which the nerves that conduct pain signals are destroyed.

Peggy noticed the television was on. "What are you watching?" she asked, trying to change the subject to something happier.

"I'm not watchin' anythin'. It's watchin' me!"

The saddest time came in the evenings when the dressings needed to be changed. No amount of pain medication could totally eradicate the pain. After a couple of such evenings, when Miss Juanita would see Peggy coming into the room with her gown on, she would say to Peggy, "It's cryin' time again!"

Afterwards, for the next thirty years, whenever a situation in the ICU required an immense amount of perseverance, such as when a patient vomited all over himself, or when a patient was incontinent and stooled from his hips to his toes, or smeared his stool on his face or sheets, we would find another nurse to help us clean up the patient, and we would say, "It's cryin' time again."

Several years after Peggy's encounter with Juanita, Nurse Darla and I were cleaning up a patient whose stool had not been contained. We turned the patient on his side on the edge of his bed and worked several minutes to do a thorough job. After finishing, we put the patient in a fresh johnny and changed his sheets. The memory of that big cleanup seemed to linger with Darla throughout the day. She smelled feces wherever she went and in whatever she did. Her lunch could not even drown out the memory. Later the same day when the phone rang, she picked it up.

"First floor ICU, Darla speaking," she answered.

Darla needed to write a message and thrust her hand into her scrub jacket pocket for her pen. Her fingers instead met with a softer, slimier resistance, and she realized with disgust she had been carrying around a pocketful of feces for several hours. She dropped the phone and tore off the jacket. "Darla, it's cryin' time again!"

"Put your hand on a hot stove for a minute, and it seems like an hour. Sit with a pretty girl for an hour, and it seems like a minute. THAT'S relativity."
~Albert Einstein

My neighbor Walter worked in road construction as one of those guys you see in the heat of summer raking hot asphalt into place on new roads. On one unfortunate day, a load of asphalt was accidentally dumped on top of him, and he suffered second-degree burns over much of his body. When he came in, he was covered with the black, sticky substance.

Seeing me, he winked and commented, "I bet you didn't know your neighbor was a n*****!"

This man's prejudicial remark took me by surprise, and I ignored it, choosing instead to concentrate on wishing him a speedy recovery.

"Sorry to see you in here. We'll get you looking like yourself again in no time."

I assigned Nurse Catherine this patient during his second day with us, and she asked me to assist in turning Walter, who weighed 580 pounds. During this procedure, one of the man's arteries, eroded by the burn, ruptured, and he bled profusely. It wasn't until after we succeeded in stabilizing Walter that we noticed blood had poured out and soaked the clothing over Catherine's lower torso, hip, and groin area. She walked out to the nursing station and began to scrub at the stains to no avail.

Accustomed to taking care of the people who took care of the people, I went to her rescue.

"Catherine, I'll get you fixed up."

She looked up from her scrubbing, not knowing how I was going to tackle so much of a mess but appreciative of the sentiment.

"I'll be right back," I continued.

I walked to the laundry facility, which was nestled in the basement of one of the oldest buildings of the medical center, and was able to secure some OR scrubs. When Catherine saw me return with these articles, her face lit up.

"These are great, but Ray, the blood soaked through my panties too."

This was beginning to get a little out of my comfort zone, but my guardian instincts persevered.

"Wait. I'll be right back."

I dialed the maternity ward.

"Seventh floor, Maternity. Can I help you?"

Usually, it takes a couple of rings to have a call answered—time to sort out what you want to say. Sometimes not.

"Uh, do you happen to have any panties," I asked, concentrating more on disguising my deep voice than on my words.

"I beg your pardon?"

"This is ICU. We have need of some mesh panties—you know, the kind you use to hold the pad for hysterectomy patients."

"Oh sure. I'll tube a pair right down."

Our pneumatic tube system was the best thing to happen to ICU since IV Propofol. (Propofol is a short-acting, intravenously-administered, hypnotic/pre-anesthetic agent, which we used to sedate patients on ventilators.) Though hospital administration eventually buckled down on what could and could not be sent interdepartmentally via this tube system, we preferred the model used by the United States Postal Service (USPS): "If it fits, it ships." We used it for sending anything that could be bundled small enough to fit into one of the tube's bullets: from dentures and money for Girl Scout cookies to some of my famous tuna noodle casserole in a bag. We had even been known to "ship our pants" on more than one occasion. Once, we misaddressed a sputum sample to the library instead of to the laboratory and waited patiently for them to "read" it. When we didn't get a result in the anticipated timeframe, we discovered it had never made it to the lab. A search was instituted by our engineering department, who determined the specimen had been "shelved" pending more information. Now the tube system was once again proving its efficacy, and the panties arrived safely via the tube system within a few minutes of my call.

Catherine was ecstatic when I brought her the mesh panties in a tube bullet bundle. In future years, whenever I asked Catherine if she could work an extra shift and whenever Christmas and her birthday came around, I told her I had an extra pair of mesh panties for her. Only on special occasions could she again get her panties in a bundle.

"We as nurses have a privilege to relieve human suffering and pain, both medicinally and emotionally."
~Author Unknown

Though we sometimes have to clean up physical messes, these are dwarfed next to the messes with which we are left when some physicians "hit and run." I am referring to the times when patients are given bad news in a cold and brief exchange from their physicians and are left to cope with it on their own. This rarely seems to happen anymore, but from time to time, we may still be confronted with such situations.

One of our social workers hobbled into my office one day, visibly upset. She was a transplant from Tijuana, Mexico, a little lady who took a maternal approach to everybody's business, and that day was no exception.

"What's wrong?" I asked, helping Lena to a chair.

"Disney."

"Disney?"

"Disney is killing me," she answered, patting her knee. "And I have a creek in my neck. I moustache you something."

"I'm all ears," I said, fingering the growth above my upper lip and focusing all my attention on Lena's forthcoming question.

"Ray," she began, "you are always totally engaged with whomever you are talking to. We have a million and one distractions in the unit, but they don't distract you from the one person who is pouring out his heart to you." She started to cry.

"Oh good. I like it when girls come into my office crying. Have a tissue. Go on, please," I said. I swept a handful of pens I had inadvertently misappropriated from staff earlier that morning into my coat pocket and handed her a box of Kleenex.

Lena's brows knit together, and she eyed me suspiciously. "Is that my pen?" she asked.

I pulled my pocket open and peered into the jumble of pens, all colors and styles. Pen thievery and the medical profession seemed to go hand in hand---with Sister Laetitia being perhaps the only exception—but I knew I hadn't been anywhere near Lena that morning. "No," I answered without flinching. "Now, what was it you wanted to see me about?"

"I can't face Mrs. Walsh in 130. Her doctor did a hit-and-run and then caught me in the hall on her retreat."

"I'll take care of it. Thanks for letting me know," I said, knowing that things were about to get a whole lot more serious.

Just the day before, Nurse Dean had commented about having to smooth things over after Dr. V (from another provider's office) told one of his patients and the patient's family members that he didn't know what was causing his vertigo and that he'd done every test there was—"except the autopsy." I could only shake my head, trying to understand such callousness.

Now, watching the social worker leave the patient's chart on my desk, I recalled that Mrs. Walsh was the gentle, middle-aged woman whose teenage son had found her passed out in the kitchen and had scooped her up in his arms and carried her to the emergency room from over two blocks away. Now I stared at the words on the magnetic resonance imaging (MRI) and laboratory reports with dread: "Esophageal cancer, stage IV; Prognosis: Poor." Things never got any easier; I just got gentler. *Some surgeons don't offer Kleenex,* I thought. *They just drop the bomb and run.*

My feet seemed like cement blocks as I walked to 130. There Mrs. Walsh sat with the proverbial deer-in-the-headlights look. Her eyes seemed fixed on something distant but frightening, and I could only imagine the frustration she was feeling after getting a medical textbook rendition of her prognosis. She would have some tough decisions to make, and she would need a helping hand. As I approached her bed, Mrs. Walsh glanced up and quickly wiped away a tear. She smoothed over the bedcovers and looked at a wooden crucifix tacked to the bulletin board near the foot of her bed. Beside it was a picture of a handsome young man, and beyond that hung a coloring book page splashed with an assortment of bright colors. From her nonverbal, I knew I would need to wait for an invitation. Gently, I took her hand in mine, pretending to take her pulse, and felt it tremble.

The silence seemed deafening and awkward, but I tried not to let it intimidate me. I knew it was a great privilege to be invited into someone's place of suffering and, considering her recent encounter with a cold and mechanical healthcare professional, she would be choosy about whom she would let in. Reflective statements and open-ended questions work well in such instances, but the specific needs are quite individualistic. Some patients open up only after I remove my professional garb; with children, I might find the best inroads by sitting on the floor with them. In this instance, the need was acute, and I felt my heart rate pick up and felt my spirit swell with the terror of what she was experiencing, as I put myself in her place and remembered my own children. My concern was real, and all of me was there as I looked into her eyes and saw fresh tears begin to well. She seemed to recognize the genuineness in my countenance and was ready to bare her soul; I was in her presence, and she was in mine. It became clear to me later that there was another, higher presence at work here, uniting our spirits and instilling trust where there had been guardedness.

"Things look pretty rough right now for you. How you are doing with it all matters a great deal to me. Would you care to talk about it with me?" She moved over and patted a spot on the bed next to her, inviting me to sit in her presence.

"I don't understand," she began slowly.

"What have you been told?"

"He just came in, woke me up, and told me flat out, 'You have esophageal cancer, and it has spread to your lymph nodes. I can do surgery on you, you can do nothing, or I can burn you up with radiation. Either way, you have 18 months. Think about it and let me know.' Then he turned and left."

"I'm so sorry. You must be in shock."

I then listened while this sweet woman poured out her thoughts and fears. She spoke of concern about her children, and I held her hand tighter when her voice broke uncontrollably. I answered what questions I could and offered some resources to help in her decisions. Somehow in those short ten minutes of interaction, my caring got communicated to her. She knew I was able to handle whatever she threw at me and I would be there for the long haul. She also knew my spirit was troubled enough to allow her to be a real person, not just a statistic, and her coping skills improved to the point of being able to make those important decisions.

It was almost eighteen months to the day when I saw Mrs. Walsh's obituary in the newspaper, and I was perplexed about how the surgeon could have been so right, yet at the same time so wrong.

"Breathe, O breathe thy loving spirit into every troubled heart."
~ Charles Wesley, cleric, hymnist, poet

"...Meeting our patients where they are makes all the difference. In a dark hour, we were the light and I assure you that patient will not soon forget this."[9]

~ Rand O'Leary, FACHE, Senior Vice President, Northern Light Health and President, Northern Light Eastern Maine Medical Center

Louisa was a very sweet woman admitted with a multiplicity of ailments. One noticeable feature was her weight, which, when determined in order to dose her correctly, strained the loading dock scales to an astounding 648 pounds. As more and more morbidly obese patients require care in a hospital setting, nurses are challenged to maintain privacy and respect and to give such patients the best of care. Bedridden for quite some time, Louisa required four nurses to turn her in bed. On one occasion, Nurse Gail ended up in the bed with the patient on top of her.

When the ICU cared for similar patients prior to Louisa's admittance, we strapped two beds together in order to make one large enough to accommodate them. In anticipation of Louisa's stay, we rented a new type of bed, one that could be tipped to assist in getting a patient out of bed. At full tilt, Louisa could place her feet on the foot of the bed, which was then lowered to the floor, allowing her to stand.

Louisa's favorite pastime was watching television, and her favorite show was *The Price Is Right.* I walked into Louisa's room one morning just as Bob Barker was calling out, "Come on down!"

"Come on down, Louisa," I echoed, beginning a full tilt of the mechanical bed.

Louisa smiled. "I'm not used to people being so nice to me," she said.

I took her hand, and we started on our daily routine of having her stand assisted for several minutes.

"I love my nurses. And some people might call me crazy, but I can't wait each day for Mary Lou and Marlene to come draw my blood. They talk to me like I'm a regular person," she said. "And the housekeepers are so friendly. It perks me up whenever Lynn, Joe, Carolyn, Carol, or Kelly come in to clean."

I beamed with pride and gratitude whenever I saw a housekeeper leaning against a mop handle, deep in conversation with a patient or family. I knew at such moments these housekeepers were ministering every bit as much as the chaplains, social workers, nurses, and doctors. It was then we ministers would begin to appreciate how marginalized these souls sometimes felt, expressing simple wishes some of us took for granted. Like the dream expressed by one obese, young fellow of simply being able to fit in the cab of an eighteen-wheeler so that he could drive one. Having worked as a janitor at the Boston Lying-in Hospital, I had the utmost respect for the hard work the housekeepers did mopping floors and cleaning toilets, and I appreciated their taking a few moments of their time to presence with those in need.

We were a team---a good team. One of the things I tried to do each day after making out the nurse/patient assignments was to write down for the housekeepers which patient rooms would be emptied for a patient procedure or because a patient was transferring to another floor. That would allow a housekeeper an opportunity when the room could be cleaned without having the patient, bed, or equipment in the way. At that moment in time, the most important person in the room was the housekeeper.

I attended a lecture discussing the aftermath of the Oklahoma City bombing of the Alfred P. Murrah Federal Building in 1995. The blast killed 168 people, aged three months to seventy-three years, injured 680 others, damaged 324 other buildings, and destroyed eighty-six vehicles. Some 665 first responders assisted in the rescue operation. Seventy people were treated at one hospital alone. During the days after the blast, twelve thousand people participated in the relief and rescue operation. Following the tragedy, one hospital worker---overcome with guilt for not being able to do more---took his own life. That person was not a doctor, nurse, or respiratory therapist, though there were many such staff there who experienced post-traumatic stress disorder (PTSD). That person was a maintenance worker, someone who felt every bit like part of the team.

Not long after her arrival in our unit, Louisa was deemed ready to undergo several procedures that it was hoped would prolong her life. Unfortunately, things did not improve, and Louisa was placed on mechanical support. Louisa's husband sat with her most evenings, until sadly, her heart gave out one cold and snowy day in February just shy of her thirty-second birthday.

Gail was horrified that Louisa did not fit on the morgue stretcher or in a shroud. The nurses gently wrapped her in two sheets, pinned them together, and Hoyer-lifted her onto a crate wagon for transport to the morgue.

During the autopsy, the attending pathologist made the decision to strip out her organs and place them in a separate large bag for conveyance. This would help with some of the weight issues during transport. A special wooden crate was made to transport her body to the funeral home, and because she would not fit in a standard hearse, the undertaker brought his all-enclosed, wide-bodied truck. When the undertaker arrived, ten of us helped to lift her body off the table and into the crate. We then carefully lifted the crate onto the funeral home's transport cart.

The pathologist handed the bag to the undertaker, and six of us, along with the body, filed into the freight elevator, which when lowered to ground level was located near a rear exit. The truck was waiting to accept Louisa just beyond this exit door. I glanced at the elevator capacity posted on the interior wall and held my breath. It would be close.

When the elevator door opened, I breathed a sigh of relief and stepped outside into the short corridor. We all gave a heave or pull on the count of three, and the transport cart lurched forward. Unfortunately, there was a gap between the floor of the elevator and the floor of the corridor, and without warning the wheels caught and the cart collapsed. Several nurses and the pathologist were still in the back of the elevator.

The undertaker, who had led the charge, said, "I'll be right back!" He quickly dropped the bag in a snowbank just outside the exit door and returned in a matter of minutes. Even with both of his hands now freed, he was not able to repair the cart due to the considerable weight lying on it. I called Patient Transport and the engineers, and twenty minutes later, we were successful in moving the crate to a new transport table for the trip to the truck.

"Hey," I said briskly to the undertaker, "I don't know what happened, but there's a dog outside who's shredding up a black plastic bag, and he's having a heck of a time strewing stuff all over the place. It's a mess out there!"

The undertaker's jaw dropped, and he flew out the door. Little did he know, I'd seen him drop off the bag and thought I would teach him a little lesson. It was right where he'd left it, but I'm fairly certain he never did that again.

"Always thank your nurse, sometimes the only one between
you and a hearse."
~Carrie Latet, author

"Two men looked through prison bars, one saw mud, and one saw stars."
~Oscar Wilde, poet

My mother-in-law, Dora, was a middle-aged mother of three when she decided she wanted to do more with her life. She enrolled in a correspondence school and finished with flying colors the preparatory courses qualifying her as a licensed practical nurse. The only thing now standing in her way was to finish the internship requirement, and she quickly secured a spot in a geriatric unit at one of the local hospitals.

She was first assigned to two gentlemen who shared the same room. Ralph was a very quiet and undemanding elderly gentleman. He would always do what he was asked by staff, never complained, and rarely needed assistance with any of his daily functions. Ralph was also blind.

In the bed next to Ralph was Henry. There could not have been a greater mismatch of roommates than these two. Henry was uncooperative, complained about every little thing, found reasons not to ever do what he was asked, and always needed assistance—not because he was unable to do things, but because he thought he should be pampered. Staff resorted to using diapers on him, since he would soil himself to punish the caregiver if his needs were not attended to immediately.

Dora had grown up in a poor family and had worked hard all of her life to get to where she was. She and her brothers and sisters had always pulled their own weight, and Henry's attitude grated on her nerves. She taught her children that God helps those who help themselves, and she had little patience for the likes of Henry.

The first day of her internship, Dora couldn't believe how quickly the morning passed. Henry kept her so busy that it was lunchtime before she could catch her breath. She handed her patient off to the registered nurse who oversaw her instruction, walked to the break room, and retrieved her deviled ham sandwich and soda from the refrigerator.

Dora had barely taken a bite when the RN appeared at the door. "Henry has messed himself and needs to be changed."

"Is it okay if I finish my lunch first?"

"Visiting hours are about to start. Sorry, but could you please help me with it now?"

Dora was used to changing her kids' diapers, but nothing could have prepared her for the unpleasantness of changing an adult. When she finished cleaning up Henry, she ducked into a nearby restroom and vomited, thinking to herself she would never eat deviled ham again.

On her fifth day, Dora brought the lunch trays in to Ralph and Henry. Ralph thanked Dora, opened his milk carton and inserted a straw, unwrapped his utensils, and began to quietly eat his meal. Henry took a fistful of peas and threw them at the wall opposite his bed. They streamed down the wall in a river of green.

"Why'd you do that?" Dora asked impatiently. She looked at Henry with disgust. She looked at Ralph, who continued to eat his meal peacefully; then she looked back at Henry.

Henry just laughed. He seemed to enjoy her discomfort and anger. He had no idea with whom he was dealing.

Dora picked up his tray, which except for the peas was untouched, and removed it to the cafeteria cart. She charted that Henry had preferred not to eat, grabbed her lunch from the break-room refrigerator, and left, vowing never to become a nurse. It takes a special tolerance to become a nurse. Some of us are cut out for it; others are not.

"...anger hath a privilege."
~William Shakespeare, *King Lear*

There are times when caregivers are confronted by patients who are angry about collateral damage that occurs during the course of trying to save their lives. Ellen tried to sue the ER because the ER staff needed to slice through her leather jacket. Her husband, Eric, was admitted after the motorcycle on which they'd both been riding crashed and slid beneath the cab of a truck. Besides incurring abdominal injuries, his perineum had been burned by the truck's exhaust system. So much for Mom's advice to make sure you have on clean undies "in case you get into an accident"! Even if the patient had arrived at the ER clothed, the famous scissors with which all ER nurses are equipped would most assuredly have come out and cut away any obstacles such as clothing rather than risk further injury to the spine by trying to remove it the conventional way. The ER staff knew Eric as a "frequent flyer," who had come in on numerous other occasions with much less serious complaints.

After several of us nurses worked on stabilizing Eric with blood transfusions, further tests revealed abdominal bleeding, which required emergency surgery. Since Eric was unconscious, Ellen gave permission for the doctors to proceed.

"Of course," she said. "Do whatever it takes to save his life."

Two doctors worked for several hours trying to stop the bleeding. When they finally emerged from the OR, they felt satisfied they'd done everything they could.

Eric would remain unconscious for the next two weeks, after which he seemed unusually anxious to get the bandages removed from his abdomen and to see his scars. When the day finally arrived, he was mortified to find the surgeons had sliced through the second word of his beloved tattoo, "Hard Rock Café," rendering the *R* now a *C*.

"Did you do your 'belongings list'?"

Nurse Karyn smiled and handed me a sheet of paper on her way to check on another patient. "Would I ever let you down, Ray?" she asked.

I peered over the rims of my glasses. "You? Never." I scanned with satisfaction the report she'd detailed, noting all the items her patient, who was being transferred to another floor, was taking with him. I matched it up against the belongings list I'd received upon his admission to the ICU and saw that nothing was missing: one shopping bag containing a pair of shoes, socks, pants, and a shirt; one shopping bag containing a watch, wedding band, framed picture of his wife and daughters, and a recent copy of *Sports Illustrated*; and a third shopping bag containing a large bag of M&M's, three hardcover novels, a book of crossword puzzles, a pair of pliers, and a box of thank-you cards.

Keeping track of the possessions of a newly admitted patient can present another challenge for nurses, as the circumstances surrounding the patient's admittance are often mired in urgency. Relocating lost articles can sometimes be a messy affair, fraught with mystery and frustration, especially since families count keeping these possessions safe as one of a nurse's biggest responsibilities.

Northern Maine is home to buckwheat ployes, potatoes, and some of the biggest snowfall totals in the country. Snow removal from housetop roofs has always presented a perilous dilemma, and some men have fallen to their deaths or endured serious injury in tackling the job. After having shingled the roof of the first house I built, I have great respect for being able to repeatedly scale such heights. On days I didn't have a babysitter and needed to keep an eye on my baby son while I was up there, my own fear of heights prompted me to nail his overalls (with him in them) to the rooftop.

Roy was barely into the third decade of his life in the northern town of Fort Kent when he ended up in our hospital, the victim of a fortuitous stumble. Having come from a poor family, "without a pot to piss in or a window to throw it out of," he'd liked going up to the rooftop, where he had a bird's-eye view of his community and could almost forget the burdens that came with being the breadwinner of his family. Now, he was gone.

Roy's wife wanted to have Roy cremated and asked a neighbor to pick up his body in his station wagon and drive it to the crematorium in Bangor. We packed up his belongings, put them in a plastic bag, and gave the bag to the driver of the station wagon.

Earlier that day, a patient from Machias had died in the room next to Roy. The undertaker came and took his body to the funeral home in Machias. At 6:00 pm I received a call from the Machias Funeral Home.

"We are planning visiting hours for him tomorrow evening, but we don't have his dentures. Can you help us recover them tonight?"

I immediately launched an investigation and spent the next two hours trying to trace the whereabouts of the missing dentures. I knew this patient hadn't been part of a multiple-casualty crash, a type of event that had resulted the previous year in dentures being switched due to delayed labeling in the double bay of the emergency room and being buried in a spouse's mouth. Remembering that Nurse Leo had once flushed dentures away in a bloody vomitus wash basin, I checked our deceased patient's chart and found no report of the patient having vomited. Experience also prompted me to call laundry to make sure a set of dentures hadn't been found in the dirty sheets. Calling each nurse and housekeeper who had come into contact with the dentures, I finally came to the conclusion the dentures had been packed into Roy's plastic bag and transported via the station wagon to the crematorium. I called Roy's wife and asked for the phone number of the station-wagon driver, fearful the dentures had been cremated with the body.

"Do you still have Roy's plastic bag of belongings, and if so, is there a set of dentures in it?" I asked the man.

"Just a minute, and I'll go look in my car." He returned a few minutes later. "Yes, to both questions," he said.

My heart jumped back into place.

I called a cab to pick up the dentures and have them delivered to the Machias Funeral Home. The tab was $175.00, but it was well worth it. The dentures arrived at midnight, in time to avoid rigor mortis from preventing placement and to make their client presentable for the following evening.

"This is a Prozac moment."
~ Anonymous

Medical centers are like little cities, complete with departments that maintain the facility's infrastructure, keep the environment clean and sanitary, regulate the flow of patients and guests, dispense life-saving drugs, handle publicity, provide nutritious meals, and a myriad of other essential, tightly coordinated tasks. The actions of one department can have a significant downstream impact on the ability of another department to fulfill its obligations. Breakdowns in coordination can lead to messy situations, the underlying cause of which are not always appreciated.

One of a nurse's many challenges involves giving medications to patients in the correct time frame. Our hospital policy called for a medication to be given no earlier than a half hour before the scheduled time and no later than a half hour after the scheduled time. At the height of a particularly frustrating period when ordered medications were not being delivered to our automated Pyxis MedStation, I thought about placing a microphone at the Pyxis station to make Pharmacy aware of the "oral frustration" spawned when drugs were not dispensed. Not only did a drug no-show require the nurse to call the pharmacy to let them know the scheduled med was not in the bin, but a third of the time the reordered drug didn't arrive in the approved time frame, prompting the nurse to then have to write an incident report. That required five minutes to reorder the drug and ten minutes to write the incident report, time that might have been used in a more patient-focused activity.

I picked up the phone and talked to Pharmacy. "We're having some issues with our meds getting here on time," I said. "Is there anything we can do to ensure better service?"

"There are two kinds of pharmacists," Pharmacy Lou answered. "Both profess the *R*s."

"The *R*s?"

"Yup. The first kind is the one who believes in giving the <u>R</u>ight medication to the <u>R</u>ight patient at the <u>R</u>ight time."

"Sounds perfect. And the second kind?"

"The second kind is the one who professes <u>R</u>ules and <u>R</u>egulations."

"Like having the appropriate requisition?"

"Yup. You see, if these pharmacists are asked to fill prescriptions written on miscellaneous charge slips instead of pharmacy slips, they're too busy to call ICU and ask for the orders to be rewritten on the appropriate slips. It would otherwise require them to transcribe the orders onto the appropriate slips before the slips are forwarded on to accounting. It's a hard lesson for the ordering departments but one which will stick if it happens to them frequently enough. Can you understand our position?"

"Yes," I said, regretting having just tubed to the lab five tubes of blood collected during a code and wrapped together with a single piece of masking tape labeled with the patient's name. I appreciated those who tweaked the rules a bit to accommodate emergency situations but also understood their position. A little in-service to our staff the following day helped address the situation by reinforcing rules and regulations so that the right medication could then get to the right patient at the right time.

Sometimes, *bending* a rule can be in everybody's best interests, as the following encounter demonstrates.

Coordinating with MRI requires that the initiating department remove anything metallic from a patient's external body. The MRI's powerful magnetic field attracts iron-containing metals and can cause serious injury or can distort the MRI image and make it difficult to read. Metal piercings, in particular, can be pulled out by the MRI, leading to injury.

When a sixteen-year-old female was transferred from Franklin County to our ICU after a cheerleading fall in which she sustained head trauma, Dr. G was called. The teen arrived intubated and sedated.

"Any family with her?" Dr. G asked.

"Her mother is coming. She should be here in about an hour," I said.

"Okay. Let's get her to MRI right away."

"The patient has several piercings, Doctor. They need to be removed first."

Dr. G consulted the patient's chart: *piercings present on both ears (three each), left eyebrow, tongue, bottom lip, bilateral nipples, naval, and clitoris.* In those days, our medical establishment preferred that piercings be removed by the attending physician. The pulmonologist loosened his necktie. "Who's her primary nurse?"

"Nurse Anna Marie," I said, just as Anna Marie entered the room.

"I'm willing to bet this gal hasn't told her mom about some of these piercings."

Anna Marie and I nodded. "I bet you're right, Doctor," Anna Marie said. "Most moms still bake 'sweet-sixteen' cakes for their daughters."

"I'm also inclined to bet, Anna Marie, that you'd be willing to remove the piercings for a price."

"Maybe." Anna Marie looked intently into Dr. G's eyes waiting for his offer. He knew it needed to be good.

Dr. G pulled a beeper from his pocket and glanced at the screen. "Darn, Ray, can I see you for a minute?"

I winked at Anna Marie and held up my pointer finger to indicate we wouldn't be long. Then I stepped out into the hall with Dr. G.

"Help me out, Ray. I'm not feeling great about having to remove all those piercings."

"Well, Anna Marie is very principled. But she's reasonable. Make her a good offer, and I bet she'd be happy to do it."

"Okay," Dr. G responded, waiting for more. "So . . ." he said, scratching his neck.

"She'd probably jump at the chance to see a Celtics game in person."

"The Celtics?"

"Yup. Of course, if you'd rather---"

"Done!" Dr. G wiped the sweat from his brow and powered on a computer in the nursing station. Not long afterward, he opened the door to the girl's room and reemerged just minutes later.

"You sure do know your nurses!" Dr. G commented, sitting back down at the computer with a great sigh of relief.

It proved to be a productive collaboration for the benefit of all parties. Anna Marie removed the piercings, the MRI was successfully performed, and the mother arrived---none the worse for her cluelessness---to find a thankful patient and physician. All three were spared any embarrassment, Anna Marie went home early to enjoy hoops, balls, and studs of a different kind, and I began making plans for a potluck to go along with the requisite pie offering Anna Marie owed me for the "referral."

Chapter 5: Traveling Dilemmas

There are times when caregivers are asked to attend to patients outside a hospital room setting. The challenges of such circumstances include keeping track of patients and their belongings, as well as adapting to available resources. Sometimes, such as when I found myself attending to the needs of a victim of near-drowning at a beach on the western coast of Florida, we are called to lend our skills without prior notice. Distractions in remote settings are more numerous, but it is more important than ever to shut them out and focus on the person in our care.

> "We were given two hands to hold, two legs to walk, two eyes to see, two ears to listen, but why only one heart? Because the other one was given to someone for us to find."
> ~Author Unknown

Dick came in for routine eye surgery at a time when major construction on the main hospital tower was going on. His wife Jane, a teacher, had made arrangements to have the time off. Because he was losing his sight due to diabetic retinopathy, Dick needed his wife's guidance in directing his steps. Now a surgery held the promise of extending his sight a few extra years.

The surgery lasted just under ninety minutes, and when Jane talked to the surgeon, she was quite satisfied all had gone well.

"You should be able to see your husband in about an hour. He has to go through the usual routine in the recovery room. Everything went well, and I think you will both be happy with the results."

"Great," said a relieved Jane. "Thanks very much."

An hour came and went almost without notice in the waiting area as Jane engrossed herself for the expected wait time in correcting student papers. She glanced at the clock and thought she would try to finish the next group she had started. Another fifteen minutes elapsed. "Perfect," she thought to herself. "I'll just flip through magazines until they call for me."

When two hours slipped by, Jane dismissed the extra wait as fallout from a very busy day for hospital staff and continued perusing the journals. Another hour later, she was starting to get a little nervous.

"It's been longer than expected," she began to explain to the receptionist, who was darting about filing charts between phone calls.

"They sometimes run a little behind, Dear," the receptionist interrupted. "I'm sure everything is fine."

Jane bit her tongue and sat back down on the nearby leather-upholstered chair that held her well-worn imprint. Beside her sat an elderly lady whose husband had gone into surgery within the last hour. She looked at Jane with huge saucers of eyes and smiled reassuringly.

When shift change arrived six hours after the surgery, Jane could take it no longer. "I'd like to check on my husband's status, please," she insisted when the receptionist's replacement looked inquiringly at her. "He's been out of surgery now for six hours." The elderly lady's eyes grew wider with that report, and she glanced quickly at the receptionist, whose jaw dropped open.

"Yes, Ma'am. What is his name, please?" And then, "I'll check with Recovery."

Stone-faced, she looked up at Jane and then at the clock. Several phone calls later, she reported, "They don't have your husband in Recovery."

"Well, where is he?" Jane fairly shouted in tears. "What have you done with my husband? How can you just lose a patient?"

"They're looking to see where he might have ended up. We'll find him."

Jane looked incredulously at the receptionist. The elderly lady, whose saucer eyes were by now dinner plates, rose to her feet and wrung her hands.

Recovery room staff, patient transporters, and department heads were put on alert that a patient was missing. Because many staff involved with Dick's recovery had left from the first shift already, it took another sixty minutes of backtracking and telephone calls to locate a transporter who remembered Dick. He apologized to management for not logging the encounter, which had occurred just prior to his being called to an emergency situation.

"Yes," he began. "I did transport this patient. Entrance to the second-floor recovery room was blocked because of the construction, and I needed to find a place for him quickly because of the trauma alert that came in this morning. I think I parked him in a little alcove on the third floor."

And there was Dick, sleeping peacefully on the transport stretcher in the little alcove on the third floor. No one had noticed him there, and no one had missed him until Jane put out her plaintive plea!

There are many checks and balances in place in hospitals to prevent just such scenarios from occurring. That this did occur underlines the importance of every employee's role in preventing adverse incidents. From the dismissive attitude of the busy first-shift receptionist to the forgetful transporter suddenly called to an emergency, the care provided was not excellent enough to avoid undue suffering for the family involved. Staff nurses would do well to remember the blame is inevitably meted out to the nurse assigned to hand the patient off after his surgery. It is the nurse's responsibility to make sure the patient gets to his intended destination. In fact, the nurse as end user of many hospital services most often gets the blame. If a pharmacy technician, for example, delivers an incorrect medication and the nurse gives it to the patient, the axe falls on the nurse. If a nurse misinterprets a doctor's order because the doctor's handwriting is illegible, it is the nurse's fault.

"It's a funny thing about life; if you refuse to accept anything but the best, you very often get it."
~W. Somerset Maugham, playwright

One of my earliest ambitions when I was growing up was to ride in one of those long, gleaming limousines I would see when my eleven brothers and sisters visited the city once a year to buy school clothes. I thought perhaps this would happen when I went to the prom, or when I got married, or when I was elected president. Not in my wildest dreams did I anticipate that my first experience riding in luxury would come as a result of caring for a patient.

During my early years working in the ICU, I was frequently involved in overseeing patients who needed to be transported long distances. Bob had suffered a stroke and required a nurse to assist on his journey home with his wife to St. Augustine, Florida. The first leg of the journey, from Bangor to Portland, Maine, took place in a limousine.

The three-hour ride was uneventful. Bob was stable, although his condition predisposed him to unexpected turns of emotion. I explained to Bob's wife that stroke patients are frequently emotionally labile, and she was able to accept his bursts of anger and sadness without fearing Bob would become physically violent.

Riding in style, I watched other cars pass us and saw drivers unsuccessfully try to peer through our tinted windows. Jubilantly, I fantasized that someone might drive up alongside us with a sign requesting Grey Poupon.

Getting seated in our airplane once we reached Portland also went off without a hitch. I led Bob to our seats in first class, and Bob's wife took a seat across the aisle, where she ignored us for the rest of the flight. It seemed she was embarrassed by Bob's lability and his clumsy movements. At one point during the flight, Bob got a little agitated, and the stewardess, unaware of the situation, asked me if I could calm my father.

"Sure," I said, "I'll quiet down my dad."

"Thank you," she said. "Now, would either of you like anything to drink?"

"I'll have a rum and coke." Bob slurred his words, but I understood what he wanted.

"No," I answered. "He's not going to have anything. Nor am I."

From this point on, Bob was even more agitated, but I did my best to pacify him and keep things from getting out of hand.

Some stroke patients have ravenous appetites, and such was the case with Bob. When my meal was served before his, he looked with such longing at it that I passed it to him. When the stewardess brought another tray for me, Bob had already finished the first tray and was looking at mine again. I ended up giving him my dessert and my milk.

Minutes later, when the "seat belts off" sign came on and I needed to take "Dad" to the bathroom, the stewardess shot me an understanding and sympathetic glance. I held Bob by his belt to steady his steps, and we would have done well had it not been for some unexpected air turbulence on our way back to our seats. The instability threw both of us off-balance. I caught hold of the seat I was passing, and Bob lunged forward, landing on his knees with his face planted squarely in the well-exposed bosom of a shapely blonde.

I was afraid Bob had passed out, because he didn't move for several seconds, but something told me he was just taking advantage of his disability.

"We're so sorry," I said to the woman, while I helped Bob to his feet.

Bob seemed calmer the rest of the flight, and his wife commented about the strange, cockeyed smile on his lips.

My protective instincts kicked in. "He's probably happy to have had his bathroom needs met."

It was another half hour's ride in a limousine from the airport in St. Augustine before I was finally able to get this prominent business executive and his sophisticated wife to a rehab center near his home. A first-class ride all the way. Once at the rehab center, however, I looked on in shock while a very large, no-nonsense nurse's aide tossed Bob onto a bed, flipped him over as if he were a piece of meat, and dressed him in his pajamas.

Maybe the nurse's aide made them appreciate me more, because, besides the limousine rides and my hourly wage, Bob and his family were so pleased with the trip that they gave me a twelve-hundred-dollar tip. I spent a week relaxing in the sun at a nearby resort before coming back to Maine with five hundred dollars left in my pocket.

Home health nurses provide an indispensable service to patients well enough to avoid nursing homes. They allow patients to be cared for in the comfort of their own homes. While in nursing school, Marcy worked first as a certified nurse assistant for a home health agency and was assigned the task of giving one such patient a bath.

When Marcy rang the doorbell, there was no answer. She rang again, and upon checking her notes and realizing Sandra lived alone, Marcy opened the door and went inside. She found Sandra lying in the living room on the couch.

"Hello," she began. "My name is Marcy, and I'll be your caregiver this afternoon. How have you been?"

"Fine," the elderly woman said. "My daughter just checked on me."

Seizing upon the opportunity to connect with her patient, Marcy launched into conversation about family. Sandra seemed tickled to have the company, and the pair conversed for a good thirty minutes.

"Well," said Marcy. "I'm going to give you a bath."

"I don't need a bath."

Marcy looked at Sandra and saw herself in the old woman's frightened, vulnerable eyes. *I'd say the same thing if this were me*, she thought to herself. She walked down the hall until she found the bathroom, where she began to prepare a wash basin and washcloths for the bath. A few minutes later, Marcy returned to the old woman's side and decided to gain more of Sandra's confidence before asking her to be bathed by someone she barely knew. Forty-five minutes passed, and Marcy knew the agency would be wondering where she was.

"Okay if I give you your bath now?" she asked.

"No, thank you."

"If you change your mind, give me a call, and I can be over in a short time."

Marcy was not about to force the situation. She smiled, put on her coat, bid farewell to Sandra, and left to see her next patient. As she drove home a few hours later, she thought about what a sweet lady Sandra was. It hadn't been a total waste of time, since she knew Sandra really enjoyed having the company. The chime of a cell phone interrupted her thoughts. It was the home health agency.

"The family of Sandra Jones just called and wondered if you could come in and bathe her now."

Marcy explained the patient's refusal. With a family member now present, a bath would not seem so intrusive, and she turned her car around. She parked on the road this time and stepped onto the asphalt driveway leading to the side door, remembering that the front door looked less used. The sun was about to set, and she shivered at the thought of winter's approach. The leaves had fallen from a pretty oak tree next door, littering the lawn with splashes of red and gold where a marker identified the address on that house as "501 Oak Lane." *How appropriate!* she thought.

And then it hit her. "501 Oak Lane" was Sandra's address. Who was the poor lady whom she had tried to talk into a bath earlier? A flushed feeling came over Marcy when she realized it was only by coincidence that the lady in *503* Oak Lane was also elderly. Whoever this woman was, Marcy felt certain she and her family would be wondering the same thing about who Marcy was and why she'd come into her home and tried to give her a bath!

"Every man has a right to a Saturday night bath."
~LBJ

99

Chapter 6: Loss

Subchapter 1: Dealing with Families: A Perceptible Difference

"As a nurse we have the opportunity to heal the heart, mind, soul, and body of our patients, their families and ourselves."
~Maya Angelou

I nevitably, the nurse must be prepared to deal with the families of patients, for it is the families from whom patients come and to whom patients usually want to return. They are the external lifeblood connected by the nurse umbilicus. We as caregivers must educate families about their loved one's condition, must answer concerns and questions related to care, and must sometimes even run interference on behalf of the patient. At all times, we must be patient advocates. Words must be chosen with care, because what is said and how it is said can have far-reaching consequences.

Sometimes families do not present as typical. Nurse Eileen had a patient who was brain dead on a ventilator. The patient's brother came in to "visit" with a supersized bag of popcorn and stood there eating it as if he were watching a movie. Another of her deceased patients, whose family was of an unconventional religion, came and collected his body in a station wagon. It's unclear what they did with it.

Familiarizing oneself with patient demographics can be helpful in preparing for the influences of different cultures in everyday life and death situations. However, because there is a wide spectrum of observance among different sects and every patient and family is different, assumptions should not be made. Good general guidelines include 1. asking the patient about cultural wishes and concerns; and 2. consulting resources, including spiritual leaders, to help with any questions you may have. Cultural and religious beliefs may influence specific activities on particular days of the week, dietary restrictions, issues of physical modesty, the administration of medications or life-saving procedures, organ donation, autopsy, end-of-life care, and death rituals, to name but a few concerns.

There is, of course, a fine line between respecting another's religious or cultural beliefs and providing the best care. We found that out the hard way early in my nursing career when Nick came into the ICU with a head injury. In the medical field, a *widow maker* refers to an occluded coronary artery (specifically, a blockage of the left anterior descending artery), which can lead to a massive heart attack and sudden death. Here in Maine, neurosurgeons also use the term when referring to a tree or part of a tree that falls on someone and causes a head injury. Lumbering is a big industry in Maine, and many men like Nick have met their fates after being struck by falling trees.

Nick's family belonged to an unorthodox religious sect which did not believe in the use of machines to keep people alive. They passionately believed God had told them their loved one would live if we disconnected him from mechanical support. This discussion continued for a couple of weeks, and they became more and more adamant in their position.

Dr. B was a new, albeit very gifted and smart, neurosurgeon from the Philippines. Though he was actually a man with an infectious laugh and a kind and gentle disposition, his broken and college-campus-influenced English, in which he often unknowingly switched pronoun genders or used popular expressions, sometimes caught families off guard and complicated the discussions. It wasn't unusual for him to address a nurse as "Baby."

"She'd all fooked up," Dr. B said to the family one day. Dr. B, of course, heard the phrase used in difficult cases but was blissfully unaware of its origin until I pulled him aside one day and enlightened him. Ten minutes after we finally gave in and disconnected the head-injured man from mechanical support, he died.

Not long afterward, an Asian woman was injured while climbing Maine's highest peak, Mt. Katahdin. Many Native Americans believe that the storm god Pomola inhabits Katahdin, and they avoid the area. Between 1933 and 2020, the mountain claimed at least sixty lives, many due to exposure in inclement weather and falls from the Knife Edge, a three-foot-wide trail extending for three tenths of a mile and dropping off precipitously on either side. Our patient, however, had the misfortune of having been struck by lightning there. We allowed the woman's sister to apply copper bracelets on the woman's wrists and ankles, but we didn't stray from our usual treatment plan for such a patient. IV drips supported her blood pressure, decreased the swelling in her head, and were used to administer antibiotics, and she was on a ventilator. Her sister, of course, was convinced the bracelets saved her life. Similarly, it has long been known that Black slave ancestors' power of healing through witchcraft lay in the *patients' belief* it would work.

In regard to running interference on the patient's behalf, one case stands out above the rest. An eighty-year-old nun was admitted with a tumor in her frontal lobe, the part of the brain responsible for managing self-control and maintaining appropriate learned social behaviors. An intact frontal lobe is what keeps people from picking their noses and wiping their fingers on the wall, from swearing in public, or from taking off their clothes and running naked in the streets. As one physician put it, the frontal lobe governs "executive" functions.

On the first morning after her admission to the ICU, the lovely nun's Mother Superior visited her. Walking through the door, she glanced at the nun's starched white wimple, sitting proudly on the windowsill at the side of her bed. A large wrap of clean white dressing on the nun's head now replaced it, covering everything from her ears up. A few wisps of fine, gray hair peeked out below the bandages in the back, and in the front, a red line ran all along her face above her brows and down the sides of her face and across her chin. This was the impression made by her wimple, worn faithfully from the time she rose until the time she retired each day for the past seventy years. Despite her age, the only lines on her face besides this one were smile lines---which framed her delicate lips---and fine crow's feet, evidence that her eyes had sealed the sincerity of joyous moments.

"What the f*** are you doing here?" the nun blurted out when her superior entered the room.

"I beg your pardon, Sister?" came the startled response.

"You aren't my sister. And take that silly thing off your head. You look like a f***ing penguin!" she added, lifting her johnny and scratching her stomach.

I entered the room to check on vitals just as the conversation was getting started and lost no time in taking the poor, red-faced Mother Superior by her elbow and leading her gently to the hall. If I'd known she was going to visit, I would have preferred to have intervened *before* this point.

"Oh, rats!" I said to myself, evoking a nurse's ability to share feelings in just a few simple words, a gesture, or even a nonverbal glance. Nurse Peggy had worked in large city hospitals and had seen lots of new, emerging diseases. In the 1980s there was acquired immune deficiency syndrome (AIDS). Peggy told us how AIDS was spread rapidly in the gay community when men declawed small rodents and put them in their rectums to stimulate their bulbocavernosus reflexes. After that, we used the phrase "Oh, rats!" when we found ourselves in a pickle. "Oh, rats!" I said again under my breath.

"I'm sorry, Mother Superior." I began to explain that her charge had no control over her social graces due to the tumor's effect on the frontal lobe.

By this time, the damage was already done. Like feathers tossed off a mountaintop, words once spoken are almost impossible to get back. Though someone with frontal lobe damage is unable to taste words before spitting them out, the unprepared Mother Superior had been assaulted emotionally, and such trauma set up an instinctual flight-or-fight response, which colored her understanding with mistrust. Undoing such damage is more difficult than preventing it. Other members of her religious family who subsequently visited were warned of these things beforehand. They were better able to dismiss them, since they were well prepared to accept that everyone has such thoughts stored from some former point in their lives and that such thoughts do not necessarily represent present feelings.

"Life is a succession of lessons which must be lived to be understood."
~Helen Keller, author

Since I'm sure the statute of limitations has run out for this, I will confess a true incident that illustrates how someone can be overwhelmed by too much information. As a twenty-one-year-old switchboard operator at the Boston Lying-in Hospital for Women, and---I might add---the first male to ever work at its switchboard, I found myself alone at the switchboard on a particularly busy evening, when normally there would have been three operators. In those days, the telephone lines consisted of two sets of cables, one for incoming calls and the other for connecting to the extensions.

On this particular night, all of the fifty or so lines at one point were connected and busy, and I suspected I had made a few wrong connections. I just couldn't imagine that on a Friday night these people didn't have anything better to do than to call and bother me. I hadn't even had a chance to pick up my copy of *Popular Mechanics*; nor had I been able to take a puff from one of my coveted Parliament cigarettes. Parliaments at the time came in a nice blue and white cardboard box, and their triangular recessed tips were heavily promoted. I could take the cigarette, create a vacuum with the tip, attach it to my lip and hold it there for as long as I needed. I thought the technique I'd developed was pretty innovative and often felt the company was losing out by not having me in one of their cool commercials.

Weighing my options for relief, I considered the possibility of an electrical storm, which might occasionally knock out the power, but such storms were not common in the dead of winter. Surely, administration would not let me call in another operator. Perhaps people were calling in just to hear my voice, which I'd been told was made for the telephone, and I briefly considered raising it a few octaves. In the end, being young and cocky and feeling overwhelmed, I made the decision to take matters into my own hands (literally). I grasped the bundle of wires and yanked every single connection, and—*poof!*—they were all gone. *Okay, call back, folks.* Only three or four calls came in after that. *See, I knew you could find something better to do on a Friday night in Boston!* After several months on this job, something had to give, and, thankfully, it was my cigarette habit that eventually went up in smoke.

This was obviously more information than I was capable of handling at one time. To avoid the same mistake my supervisor made in leaving me alone so soon, good charge nurses should evaluate what their nurses are capable of and encourage them to speak to families in increasingly more complex circumstances. Much is at stake for all concerned. As a charge nurse, I always felt my primary job was to take care of the people who take care of the people. And I was never afraid to show the other nurses that I was not above doing anything I would ask *them* to do. Whenever there was a spill that required mopping up, for instance, I tried to be the first one to the housekeeping closet to retrieve and start using a mop. In fact, at a time when there were lots of vice presidents in the hospital and it seemed as if those with the longest titles had the least important jobs, I dubbed myself *vice president of the mops.* I held a great deal of respect for the maids and janitors, perhaps because my first job other than switchboard operator at a hospital was that of janitor.

After several months as a switchboard operator, I learned to think ahead. This had both good and bad consequences. It greatly improved my reflexes in placing the telephone wires, but the tendency to jump from the present to the next step became hard-wired and followed me into nursing. Thinking ahead was great in circumstances in which anticipating the next action quickly was advantageous, such as knowing what to do in emergency situations. But I needed to learn that families require time to digest what has happened before jumping to the next step. When my daughter died, for example, I was already talking about funeral preparations, while the rest of the family was still trying to come to terms with her death. Just as I had been overcome with too much information as a rookie switchboard operator, family members in acute emotional distress are usually short on the necessary resources for making long-term decisions.

A wise person once described an *expert* as one who has made more mistakes than others. An elderly woman in my care was rendered in a vegetative state. Two years prior to her admission, her son had unexpectedly died. Every day after his death, she visited his grave, crying her eyes out, until one day she tried to end her sorrow with carbon monoxide. A month after she was admitted, I asked the grieving husband if he planned to put his wife in a nursing home. Because he was still hopeful for a recovery and needed more time to process the situation, he was very angry about my asking this. How much kinder it would have been to have waited for this man to open a door of opportunity through which I could then have advanced such a question! I learned through experience that I needed to let families deal with circumstances in their own time frames and to wait for that invitation.

As defined in the introduction along with key components, presencing is not a right, but a privilege, and can take place only at the invitation of the person who is suffering. In the words of oncology and grief crisis counselor, Jan Pettigrew, PhD, RN,

> Nothing apart from the permission or invitation of the other person ever gives the nurse the right to enter another's pain, whether it be physical, emotional, relational, or spiritual. The invitation is to come alongside and be allowed to see, to share, to touch, and to hear the brokenness, vulnerability, and suffering of another. Because the cost of exposing one's suffering, woundedness, and grief is extremely high, presence is always regarded and approached with great humility as a gift and a privilege.[6]

Thus, armed with the hard lessons of experience, I arrived in the heat of the summer of 1990, when an opportunity for teaching one of our new young nurses arose. A sudden storm had swept a father, mother, and son into a nightmarish fight for their lives after capsizing their fourteen-foot motorboat in the middle of great and turbulent Moosehead Lake. The father sustained non-life-threatening injuries, and the mother's injuries

107

were serious enough to warrant keeping her in ICU. The son, unfortunately, did not survive. I asked rookie Nurse Brooke if she would be willing to care for this family. I knew Brooke could adapt and would be willing to do what I asked. Our plan was to put both parents in the same room and to bring the boy from the morgue so that the parents could see him one last time.

"I've never done anything like this before," Brooke said.

"I know you are not very confident in your personal life. But when you step over the threshold into the patient's room, I see your confidence as a nurse. I know you can do this," I reassured her. "You won't have any other patients today, and the father won't require much help. We'll do this together."

Over the next hour, we moved the father into the mother's room and gave them some time to come to terms together with their terrible loss. When they were ready, we brought the young boy from the morgue on a stretcher and wheeled him into the room with his parents. The couple spent the next four hours saying goodbye, while we stood ready to assist them with anything they might need.

The following day, a Catholic priest went in to visit with the couple.

"He's in a better place," he told the grieving mother.

"Get out of my room! Don't you tell me he's in a better place!" the mother sobbed.

The priest, who apparently also needed to learn this hard lesson, left quickly.

Meanwhile, the father's neighbor found me in the nursing station.

"I don't like you talking to my friend like I heard you doing today. Please don't do it again."

He had been in the room when I talked to the father about how the room arrangements were working out and how he was coping with all that had happened. I had also told him about my daughter's death because, as Jan Pettigrew, PhD, RN put it, ". . . vulnerability demands vulnerability in order to come alongside one who is suffering."[6] Losing someone can be an isolating event because many people are afraid to talk to you and because they really cannot understand what you are going through. I quickly forgave the neighbor's sentiments and chalked it up to lack of experience in such matters. It wasn't worth arguing about. I just waited until he wasn't around and continued to do what we nurses do well. Someday, I knew, he would understand.

> "If you know someone who has lost a child, and you're afraid to mention them because you think you might make them sad by reminding them that they died---you're not reminding them. They didn't forget they died. What you're reminding them of is that you remembered that they lived, and that is a great gift."
> ~Elizabeth Edwards, attorney, author

> "It is always darkest just before the day dawneth."
> ~Thomas Fuller, author

As nurses, we are trained to attend not only to the physical and emotional needs of the patient, but also to those of the patient's family members. Part of our responsibility involves keeping healthy those to whom patient care will be entrusted when the patient leaves us. Each individual of a family brings a piece of what he or she can offer to help a patient, and it lies with us to help such individuals come up with coping strategies they will be able to use the rest of their lives. We are trained to notice whether a family member may be sleeping or eating too little or too much. We must also be attuned to listen to not only *what* a family member is saying but also *how* it is being said.

We can provide ideas and suggestions. In order for us to be there for them, it is also important to recognize *our* sadness and to deal with our own issues and conflicts as they arise, one at a time. Otherwise, we may find ourselves overcome from pent-up losses. Try to keep things in a positive light if possible. The other side of an unforgiving God, for example, is a loving God. Make sure a religious leader who will be visiting totally understands the long-term ramifications of the patient's condition, so that his words are appropriate to the circumstances.

Be creative in looking for available personal support systems. Mobilize the extended family, but be careful to find out how receptive patients are to non-family support. Beyond everything else, let them know you are there, willing and able to assist them on their terms.

There are times when a loved one is claimed not by death, but by a brain injury that renders the individual very different from the one the family previously knew. It has been widely shown that such loss involves many of the same stages of grief as are seen with death.

The first phase has been described as one in which family members may feel panic, alarm, and physical or emotional distress. They may feel powerless and scared. This is how we most often find family members immediately after a traumatic event has landed a loved one in the hospital.

In the summer of 1982, I was asked for assistance in the case of a young logger, Cliff, who had been electrocuted while attempting to secure his truck's load with a heavy steel cable. On its upswing, one end of the chain had hit the overhead high-voltage power line while the other end was held securely in his grip. As he suddenly lurched forward, his head was also zapped. Upwards of twenty thousand volts of electricity

110

entered his body through his head and hand and flowed out through his feet, severely burning the connective circuitry of nerves leading to those extremities.

I agreed to accompany him on a National Guard helicopter to Massachusetts General Hospital's ICU in Boston. While preparing for the trip, his mother, who was obviously shaken and distressed, approached me.

"Boston seems better able to handle this, don't you think? Can I ride with you?" she pleaded.

"Boston is topnotch in such cases," I said, trying to put her mind at ease. "We're flying with the National Guard, so it'll be their decision whether or not you can fly with us, but I can ask for you."

"Thanks," she said. She was obviously relieved with having these simple needs communicated. It was all she could handle in those first few terrible hours. Little things, things that seem clear-cut and simple to some of us, such as helping with decisions, can mean a lot to those so overpowered by emotional turmoil that they are unable to concentrate or process information.

As it turned out, Cliff's mother was asked to follow us on land, and she left several hours before the helicopter. Once Cliff was stabilized and loaded onto the aircraft and the pilot and I were strapped in, I felt it necessary to ask whether the patient should have the same kind of headset the rest of us did for muting the noise of the loud engine and was told in short order one was being secured for him. I heard the whirr of the helicopter blades above us and saw a man in military garb on the tarmac outside the aircraft, someone I thought would be directing the takeoff. I looked right and then left and noticed both doors were still open. *Man, we're gonna fly right outta this machine*, I thought, while visions of our patient still strapped to the gurney and falling out of the sky began to fill my head. *What's wrong with these guys?* I tapped the pilot on the shoulder.

111

"Hey, you forgot to close the doors," I said, confident I was averting a disaster.

The pilot looked back at me and smiled, while the copilot boarded, shut the doors, and buckled in. A conscientious objector, I was not familiar with military operations. Otherwise, I would have realized there are rigorous checklists preceding actions such as liftoff. I slumped back into my seat and decided to give all my attention to the patient. The military guys could handle the rest.

Monitoring Cliff's condition was critical. In those days, the aircrafts we used were not outfitted with the same equipment found in today's medical aircraft. All we carried were the monitoring equipment and some medications, so, as a precaution, we flew over towns where there were hospitals. In the event of an emergency, we could then have stopped at one of those hospitals for assistance.

Upon reaching our Boston destination and getting the patient stabilized in the ICU, I decided to use the few hours of the Guard's layover to wait for the mother's arrival and to answer any questions she might have before making the return trip back to Maine. I thought about the nontechnical terms I would use to accurately and truthfully describe his condition to a distraught mother with few available coping tools. There was an antiquated feel to the hospital, and I felt it was important to support her decision to have her son transferred there. The ICU was on the tenth floor of the building and would surely offer a magnificent view of the city.

"Look," I said to her when she walked into the room. Ushering her toward the window and doing my best impression of Vanna White unveiling letters on a giant screen, I drew open the curtains. "He's got a great view while he recuperates."

We both looked with shock at the brick wall on the other side of the glass window. The mother was not amused, and I made a mental note to check things out in advance next time.

Panic is often followed by a second stage, described as *searching behavior*, during which family members want to be surrounded by items reminding them of what they have lost. Family members are not ready to accept anything less than having the patient come back the same as he was before. In a way, it allows one to deny what has happened. When a patient or family denies a situation, it is a defense mechanism born of an inability to cope. Complex problems require complex processes, which necessarily take time, and acceptance proceeds in little pieces. Nurses who take the time can help a family to cope, which in turn helps the patient to cope. Saving answering machine messages or wearing a loved one's clothing are common examples of trying to hang on to the past.

In Cliff's case, his mother continued to make appointments on her son's behalf. She entered him in tennis tournaments, in which he had been very active, and she showered him with gifts for his twentieth birthday: a new pair of Nikes and a new Wilson racket. After two months in Boston, the young man was transferred to a rehabilitation unit nearer his home in Dover-Foxcroft, Maine.

Bridging to the third phase of mitigation may be very emotionally charged, for it represents a stage of acceptance. During mitigation, there is a 180-degree turnaround from the previous phase. Family members do not want to be reminded of what has happened and will go out of their way to avoid things or events that are such reminders. During this phase, family members often feel they need permission to not come to visit their loved one in the hospital. They have a desire to pack up their loved one's things and dispose of them. It is prudent to recognize this phase and to suggest they may want to pack it all up and put it out of sight without disposing of it. Otherwise, when this phase has passed, they may experience another loss, when they wish they had kept some of these items.

After ten months of intensive physical therapy and a physician's prognosis that Cliff would not likely improve much beyond his current condition, he and his mother came into our unit and asked if any of the teens in Pediatrics could use his old sports equipment. I looked in the boxes she had packed and carted in. There were tennis rackets, a baseball glove and bat, a football, and a Frisbee. There were also trophies from tournaments in which Cliff had participated, and he watched silently while we pawed through his treasures.

"You may want to put these boxes away for a couple of years," I suggested to his mother. "They're all packed up, so maybe you could just put them out of sight. You may want to wait before doing something rash during this transition period. If you still feel the same way in a few years, we'd be delighted to help find a good home for your son's things."

According to psychiatrist Viktor E. Frankl[10], one's ability to achieve life goals has a great impact on mental health. A patient who has suffered a head injury may feel somehow diminished in his capacity to find meaning in his life. As much as possible within the confines of a patient's particular limitations, we should encourage him to fulfill the dreams he may have laid to rest. There may be some things he can no longer do, but encourage him to focus on the things which he can still do.

"Cliff," I added. "You look much better than the last time I saw you. Have you thought about how you might continue to use your talents?"

He looked at me incredulously, as if I'd given him permission to live.

"No," he said. But I could see the wheels were already starting to turn. His mother, who seemed quite surprised, thanked me and quickly left.

The fourth phase is one of anger and of guilt. This stage can be very explosive. Anxiety and frustration must be vented somewhere, and these feelings often turn to blame. Healthcare workers, surrounded by the best modern technology can offer, are not able to heal the loved one and often get the brunt of the anger. In the minds of a loved one's family, it must be a nurse's or a doctor's choice or lack of concern that is preventing the loved one's recovery. I've found it's a good idea to step back, allow them to scream, and try to see where the emotion is coming from. Ironically, it is often the most trusted caregiver who gets the brunt of the anger, because the family member feels that person will keep coming back despite the anger. Other targets of blame include the driver of a vehicle (if the trauma resulted from a motor vehicle crash) or sometimes even the patient himself. A family member may feel irrational anger toward the loved one for not being able to do what he or she could previously do. A few years after Cliff's accident, I read in the local newspaper that his mother was suing the lumber company, alleging lack of safety equipment as a contributing factor in her son's ordeal.

Be aware also that the waiting room to a unit such as the ICU is often a boiling pot of families who have been making comparisons of their loved ones' progress and have been making determinations of the expertise of the caregivers involved. Many times, I would be approached by the receptionist in the waiting room, who would relate to me that one family was feeling their loved one was not receiving the kind of care another was, based upon their loved one's progress. Reassurance comes in the form of explaining that no two injuries and individuals are the same, and recovery can be complicated by many factors outside the control of the caregivers.

The second part of this stage, guilt, arises in family members who feel they failed to protect their loved one. They may also feel guilty for feeling jealous about someone else getting better when their loved one is not. Both of these represent feelings that linger with family members, and the best we as nurses can do for them is to validate the feelings.

The final phase is adjustment to the new reality and development of a new identity. The family member has resolved other feelings and feels a right to move on and to feel happy again. Of course, triggers lie in wait around every corner to trip up the effort and start the process all over again. The date when the loved one *should* have graduated rolls around, or one hears of the loved one's friends graduating, while the loved one has not and will not achieve this milestone. In this respect, some feel this final phase is never fully and finally achieved.

According to Nancy O'Connor (*Letting Go with Love: The Grieving Process*)[11], the degree to which any one of these phases is experienced depends on many factors, including the relationship and the degree of emotional bond an individual enjoyed with the patient prior to the traumatic event. Every family is unique, and we must not assume blood is always thicker than water. A friend may have a deeper relationship than a brother, for example.

The impact also depends upon the person's armature of coping skills. How did he previously manage losses, and what worked for him in the past in being able to cope? Engage family members in conversations about what worked for them in such instances in the past.

The amount of time one has to prepare for a loss also contributes to one's ability to cope. A chronic condition, such as cancer, gives one more time to prepare emotionally and to be ready on some level for the inevitable. An acute event, on the other hand, is much more likely to result in a family member who is out of control.

As nurses, we may do our best to prepare for the phases outlined above in attempts to heal our patients and their families and then send them on their way, only to then lose track of these precious lives. It's always uplifting when we can cross paths later and learn that somewhere between panic and acceptance, we were able in some small way to make a difference in their lives.

Twenty years after the accident, I ran into Cliff and his mother having dinner at one of my favorite fried-clam eateries in Dexter. They seemed to have adjusted well to Cliff's loss of manual dexterity and to his forgetfulness. Cliff still lived with her, helping her with the plowing and the mowing and other chores requiring strength, while his mother

116

provided him with the comforts of home. We talked for several minutes about his letting go of dreams to be a tennis pro and his transition into a new passion, one of teaching others about the sport.

"One more thing, Ray," Cliff said, as we said our goodbyes. "Thanks for closing the doors."

> "When one door closes, another opens; but we often look
> so long and so regretfully upon the closed door that we do
> not see the one that has opened for us."
> ~Alexander Graham Bell, inventor

For me, the following encounter represents a turning point in my ministry to care for patients, and I consider it the pinnacle of my career. What happened over the course of a week has never been shared with a coworker. Nor was what happened planned; there is seldom a way to predict a patient's or a family's particular needs, and there is no script one can keep handy for such interactions. Instead, one must learn to bend with the unpredictable and to be ready for whatever happens in the moment. What I did start out with was an investment of my total self, a keen awareness of the awesome privilege that I could be there in a meaningful way to someone, and a faith that my God would help direct my steps and infuse His healing power.

Forgive comes from a Greek word that means to "hurl away."

She lay alone in the room. Around her the machines swooshed and beat out a steady rhythm while neon green lines danced on the monitor. The closed blinds shut out the rest of the world while this mother lay dying.

I pushed the door open wider, quietly stepped inside and sat down beside her, lifted her hand, and held it between my own. She opened her eyes and smiled at me.

"You again," she said.

"Yes, me again. I have a question for you, if you don't mind."

"Go on."

"Your history says you have children. Can you tell me more?"

She hesitated, looked across to the other side of the room and then down at her covers. "Delila was my first. She knows where I am—quite busy with her own daughter, you know. There's not much else to tell. I have a son too, but he went away about twenty years ago, and I haven't seen or heard from him since."

"Would you like to see him again?"

"Of course. I love him. Even if he doesn't love me. But I don't know where he is or even if he is still alive." The monitor was telling me this was beginning to be too much for Jenny, and I backed off.

"May I get you a warmer blanket before I leave for the night?"

"That would be nice. Thank you."

As she turned her head and closed her eyes, a tear trickled down her pale cheek, and I promised myself I would find this wayward son before it was too late for Jenny or her son. Words of a favorite poem kept running through my mind, urging me forward in my pursuit:

Love Me Now

If you are ever going to love me,
Love me now, while I can know
The sweet and tender feelings
Which from true affection flow.
Love me now
While I am living.

Do not wait until I'm gone
And then have it chiseled in marble,
Sweet words on ice-cold stone.
If you have tender thoughts of me,
Please tell me now.
If you wait until I'm sleeping,
Never to awaken,
There will be death between us,
And I won't hear you then.
So if you love me, even a little bit,
Let me know it while I'm living
So I can treasure it.
~ Author unknown

The next morning Jenny was comatose and on a ventilator. I got report about her condition before seeing her and hesitated before entering her room. "This just isn't right," I mumbled to myself. Pushing the door all the way open, I was startled to see a heavyset woman sitting in the corner of the room reading from a Bible to Jenny. A wooden cane leaned against the arm of her chair.

"Hello," I began. "I'm glad to see Jenny has a family member who can be with her at this time."

"Oh, I'm not family. Name's Rhonda. Jenny and I have been friends since kindergarten---almost seventy-two years ago! I reckon I'm as much 'family' as anyone else she has---that's for sure. I'm guessing you haven't seen Ronnie yet, have you?"

There was a rule about admitting only family members in such circumstances, but I quickly dismissed it in this case.

"Ronnie?"

I walked to Jenny's bed. "Good morning, Jenny. It's Ray. I'm so glad I could come back and take care of you again today." I took note of

119

her vital signs, then came and sat next to Rhonda. "No, is Ronnie her son?"

"No, Ronnie is Jenny's husband. He's having a hard time with all of this. Took him by surprise, you know. One moment she was out picking green beans, and the next he was told to prepare for her death."

"She seems like such a gentle woman."

"Oh, that she is. And kind. Why, whenever people we knew died, she always made herself available. She would go into their homes and take over whatever needed to be done. Not in a rough way, mind you. But in her gentle, unassuming way, she would cook and clean and, well, just help with whatever."

Just then, the door swung open, and a balding man with a red face, a protuberant belly, and sparkling blue eyes removed his hat and stood at the foot of Jenny's bed. "I had a bad feelin' 'bout bringin' you here," he said to Jenny, nodding his head and eyeing the multitude of lines and wires leading to and from her body. "Just like that other hospital. They're all the same. Just meat factories, they are!" The man's voice rose precipitously, and I stood to try and calm him.

"Hello," I began. "Can I help you---"

"Damned right you can help me! Start by tellin' me why my wife's not sittin' up talkin' to me. You can start by tellin' me why her doctor just asked me if I wanted to give him permission not to resuscitate my wife. This is a hospital, not a funeral home, isn't it?"

"Please, let me . . ." My words trailed off, lost in exhaust fumes as Ronnie put his cap back on and stormed out of the room. Finding humility and understanding in every encounter had always been one of my goals, and I turned back to look at Rhonda, who just sat staring at the floor, biting her lower lip.

"Ronnie?" I asked.

"Yes."

"Seems like he's distrustful of the medical community. Can you tell me about other family members and how you think they might be coping?"

"That's funny. Jenny always told me I needed to be strong, but I always told her I could never be strong like her. Guess we're gonna find out. Well, now, let's see. There's a daughter, Delila, and granddaughter, Haley. I think she's fifteen. And there's a son, but . . ."

"Go on."

"It's such a sad thing," she said, shaking her head slowly and looking at Jenny's limp body in the hospital bed. She looked down at her lap, bit her lip and continued. "Jack went away many years ago. They'd had some kind of disagreement---I can't even remember what it was all about, something stupid probably. Anyway, he apparently told her he never wanted to see her again. She blamed herself and she's grieved all these years thinking she'd failed him. I heard from a mutual friend that he ended up in Farmington doing construction. So, so sad . . ."

"Yes, it is." As I checked Jenny's vitals again and drew her covers higher, Jenny's daughter Delila came into the room. I introduced myself and assured both women I would walk them through what to expect in the next few days and would answer questions related to any decisions that would have to be made. Delila sobbed uncontrollably at the sight of her mother, and I recalled how it had felt to see my own mother dying. Before I could offer any solace, Delila left the room abruptly.

"Jenny seems like the opposite of her husband and daughter," I commented.

"Yes, like two peas in a pod, Delila and her father are. Jenny always accepted Ronnie for the way he is. They've been married thirty-nine years. He's never so much as cooked an egg---well, maybe a potato. It'll be hard for him."

"Thank you for helping me to understand the family," I said to Rhonda.

121

Upon leaving Jenny's room, I found Delila in the waiting room texting to her daughter and sat down next to her.

"I can arrange for your daughter to visit her grandmother, if you'd like," I said.

Delila looked across the room and spoke as if she were talking to the walls there. "She keeps telling me she wants to see Gramma, but I'm afraid Haley would react badly to all those wires and things you got Ma hooked up to."

"How about if we took a picture of your mother and showed it to your daughter first, to kind of get her used to the stuff?"

Delila let this thought marinate several minutes and then for the first time made eye contact with me. "That sounds like a good idea. I can bring her in tomorrow afternoon." I knew time was running out but felt confident we could keep Jenny going for at least the next twenty-four hours and agreed to have a photograph available. Before retrieving the camera, I sprinted to the front desk and asked for the Farmington phonebook. How many people with that name could there be in Farmington? Only one, as luck would have it.

"Hello," the voice on the other end answered.

"I'm looking for Jack ---."

"Speaking." I should have gone out and purchased a lottery ticket. This was too easy. But after introducing myself, I knew it was about to get much more difficult.

"My name is Ray. I'm sorry to say your mother has suffered a cerebral aneurysm. A blood vessel in her head has burst. Unfortunately, she is not expected to survive."

Silence. For several seconds that seemed like minutes. "Hello?"

"I'm here."

"Your mother is dying, and I thought it would be important for you to come and talk to her. If you do decide to come, please come and see me first."

It's always difficult to predict the times when such interventions might be successful. Many times, there are extenuating circumstances of which the nurse is unaware and which prevent the ideal from being realized. Most often when the relative has little to say, as was the case with Jack, we never hear from the person again. It was with a great deal of surprise, then, that I found Jack in the waiting room when I arrived for work the next morning.

I shook his hand and thanked him for coming. He was a big, burly man in his late thirties with a ruddy complexion and large, calloused hands, but his cold, weak grasp exposed the fear within.

"I never got the chance to be gentle with my mother," he said.

"You have a chance now. Your mother is comatose. She's negotiating with her God during this time. But she can hear you. She told me she wished she could see you again. She hoped for reconciliation. And she told me she loved you. Please follow me if you're ready."

Jack flinched, trying to hold back his emotions. When I opened her door again, he walked slowly to her bedside, removed his hat, and sat down beside his mother. Before closing the door to leave them alone, I noticed the large shoulders begin to heave. He stood, bent over her still frame, kissed her forehead, and wept uncontrollably.

I also noticed Rhonda in the room and motioned to her to come talk to me. "Would you mind if Jack spends a little time alone with his mother? I think it might be a healing experience for them."

"Of course," she said.

Later, I listened at the door to check on things, and I could hear Jack talking, pouring his heart out with words he'd saved up for the past twenty years. Words of regret and words of love, they all poured out. He told of the grandchildren she would never know, of the little hands that would never hold hers, of the songs she'd sung to him and that he now sang to his own children. He told of the log cabin he'd built in the birches, of the picture of the man and woman which hung over the fireplace, of the lie about this couple's death he had told his wife to avoid the awkwardness and vulnerability of reconciliation. Some of his words to this day are powerful reminders of the ruthlessness of regret:

"Remember the night I borrowed your new car and put a dent in the hood? I thought you'd ground me, but you didn't. You just hugged me and said you were glad I was okay. And the time I knocked your casserole to the floor, saying you could *not* accompany me to the school banquet? I thought you'd keep me home that night, but you didn't. How 'bout the time you caught me smoking cigars in the attic? I thought you'd disown me then. But you didn't. And remember the time I sneaked out of my room, rode my bike into town, and stayed out till the next morning? I thought you'd tell me what an inconsiderate little prick I was. But you didn't."

After several minutes of silence, he added, "There were lots of things you didn't do, Mom. But you kept loving me through it all, and you gave me room to grow while you kept me safe. I wanted to make up the time I lost with you when you get out of the hospital . . . But you won't."

After forty-five minutes, I went into Jenny's room to check on them. "Is there anything I can do for you? Do you have any questions I might be able to answer?"

"No," Jack simply said, tears streaming down his face and his mother's hand in his own.

It has been my experience that acceptance is hindered and grief is complicated when a person's relationship with the deceased has been colored in discord and conflict. That Jack and his mother had a chance to unburden some of this strife was a precious opportunity for both of them.

Just before the body dies, there is a natural epinephrine response, which results in the elevation of vital signs. This is part of the *fight or flight response*, when the body pulls out all stops to try and prevent the inevitable, and the brain dies. Jenny's vital signs elevated at 11:00 am, and it was now almost 2:00 pm. After a brief examination of vital signs, the attending physician ordered a xenon scan and electroencephalogram (EEG), signaling his belief that brain death was imminent.

"If you have the strength, could you allow your father to come into the room with you and your mother?" I asked Jack. "It would be a healing experience for you all to be together at this time."

Jack hesitated before wiping his face with his sleeve and nodding.

I called Ronnie into the room, closed the door, and stood outside waiting for the miracle of reconciliation and love to take over. Instead, a feeling of dread and fear enveloped me when Ronnie began yelling loudly at his son. *What a crazy thing I've done! This is not at all how I envisioned it all going down.* I walked to the waiting room and consulted Rhonda.

"Well," she said. "Ronnie gets riled up easy. He usually calms down once he knows he's made his point."

I passed the photograph I'd taken of Jenny to Rhonda and allowed myself a moment of calmness. Rhonda seemed to be right. After a while, the voices softened. When Ronnie emerged forty minutes later, he sought me out. I didn't know whether to turn and flee or to call Security.

"That was the best thing that could ever have happened," he said, my confidence again beginning to rise. "It's too bad it had to wait for something like this." Gone was the angry man I'd first encountered; in his place stood a softer, calmer version. It was as if a force that filled his sails had blown itself out, and he was left alone in calm, still waters.

When Haley felt she was prepared enough by the picture to see her grandmother, she went in with Delila to see Jenny.

"Mom," she cried, "tell her to wake up!"

Several minutes later, when they returned to the waiting room, I pulled Delila aside. "Do you think Haley would like to remember her grandmother without all the tubes and wires?"

"Yes, I do. She doesn't seem able to associate the person in the bed with her Gramma."

I knew that once the results of negative brain activity came back the following day, the tubes and wires could be pulled out and still leave Jenny going for five to fifteen minutes of goodbyes. Because she wasn't an organ donor, no drugs could be administered to prolong the process. With Jenny's blood pressure dipping dangerously low in the sixties the next morning, I turned down the lights, put on some soft and easy-listening music, disconnected all the tubes and wires except for the ventilation tube, and ushered the family back in for one last visit. The only one absent was Ronnie, who said he couldn't watch Jenny draw her last breath. Having held such vigils with other families many times before this, I knew that having boxes of tissues near the bed and having the bed rail in the *down* position would be helpful, and I made sure these things were done.

With everything in place, I knew my presence with Jenny was about to end; my presence with her family would need to be stronger than ever. Standing at the back of the room, I looked into each of their faces and felt their sorrow tear at my heart: nearly thirty years of braiding hair, baking cookies, singing songs, and teaching right from wrong; more than seventy years of holding hands and sharing secrets. My body seemed to disappear as I watched it all, it seemed, from a vantage point in the ceiling. It was surreal. When I finally removed the ventilation tube and Jenny drew her last breath, a voice materialized from the radio that seemed to echo words Jenny might have spoken to those of us mourning her loss:

It doesn't mean much;
it doesn't mean anything at all.
The life I've left behind me
is a cold room.
I crossed the last line
from where I can't return,
where every step I took in faith
betrayed me
and led me from my home.

And sweet,
sweet surrender
is all I have to give.

You take me in,
no questions asked;
you strip away the ugliness
that surrounds me.
Are you an angel?
Am I already that gone?
I only hope
that I won't disappoint you
when I'm down here
on my knees.

And sweet,
Sweet,
sweet surrender
is all that I have to give.

And I don't understand;
by the touch of your hand
I would be the one to fall.

I miss the little things.
Oh, I miss everything.

It doesn't mean much;
it doesn't mean anything at all.
The life I left behind me
is a cold room.
  ~ Sarah McLachlan (*Sweet Surrender*)

The confirming neurologist came and left almost imperceptibly, slightly nodding at me on his way out.

"Your Mom died at 2:15 pm," I said to the family. "She died as peacefully as she lived her life. It was a perfect way for someone to die."

In order to help people accept their loved one's death and its finality, we must use the word *died*, not *passed* or *asleep*. And just as it is important for family to know what time someone was born, they also want to remember what time a family member died.

The last person to leave the room was Rhonda. When I tried to shake her hand, she hugged me instead for a long time.

"I couldn't have done this without you," she said.

"Thank you for helping me to understand the family," I repeated.

Putting her hand on my forehead, she said, "Give him love and give him peace."

"Be strong," I responded.

Little did Jenny's family realize that while I had been attending to their needs, a second critically ill patient in the ICU to whom I'd been assigned also depended on me to address his needs. The responsibilities nurses must manage with one hundred percent accuracy are becoming more and more challenging as hospital budgets become tighter and staffing suffers.

Before I went home that evening, Jack thanked me for letting him know about his mother. Delila also thanked me and added, "You are a wonderful man." I wouldn't know just how grateful they were until a few days later at Jenny's funeral.

The little church in Newport was packed. I didn't know why I should have attended, but I just knew I wanted to. Not expecting a great crowd, I arrived late and found myself at the very back of the church. During the service, I discovered Jenny had been a high school teacher and was beloved by her students, many of whom were in attendance. Her friend of seventy-two years, Rhonda, was also present, as were Jack and his family. I was surprised and humbled when the minister spoke of the guardian angel "Ray," whom God had sent to help the family. When I went up to receive communion, I passed the family and heard them break out into sobs. Turning to go back to my seat, Ronnie reached out and grasped my hand tightly for what seemed like several minutes before allowing me to return to my seat. God had given me the most awesome privilege in helping Jenny pass from this life.

During the reception in the church basement, I felt a tap on the back of my shoulder and turned around. It was Rhonda, and tears shone in her eyes.

"I knew you would come. When you came into her room that day and said 'good morning' to Jenny and attended so gently and with such care to her and then came and talked to me, I knew God had something great planned and everything would be okay. Because of what you did with Jenny and Jack and Ronnie, I felt we were not alone in what we were going through. I felt like Jenny had an advocate, and I just knew we were going to be okay. I prayed God would bring you here, and He didn't let me down." Then Rhonda leaned forward, gently kissed my

129

hand, and added, "I will never forget you." Her words sent chills down my spine, as I remembered the persistent urge that drove me to attend this service, something I'd done only once before, when the patient had been the close relative of a coworker.

When the funeral procession was leaving the church, Jack spotted me in the back and, wading his way through the throng, finally stood before me. "Thank you so much. You'll never know what this has all meant to me," he said, embracing me in a tearful hug.

"I'm glad it all worked out," I said, certain Jenny was at peace too, and knowing that through my presence this family had caught a glimpse of a far greater presence that would continue to sustain them long after I left.

"It isn't the burdens of today that drive men mad, but rather regret over yesterday."
~Robert Hastings

After working years in critical care, I've come to realize that what is a priority to me in caring for my patients is completely different from what is important to the family. Before visiting hours, I will have taken the patient to CT scan, changed the chest tube dressings, and resolved some oxygenation issues. I will have eight drips hanging, three of which I'm titrating, and be infusing blood. But when that family walks in the room, the first thing they will notice is that I washed and combed their loved one's hair---they will be confident that they are getting the best nursing care ever.
~Jennifer Eagle Payan, RN

The phone rang at quarter past twelve. It was Nurse Tracey calling from the first floor ICU.

"Hi Ray. Could you do me a favor and bring my lunch downstairs when you come for your meeting?"

Most people with whom I worked knew I didn't bring my lunch because I didn't want to be seen carrying a little bag or a lunchbox or *girlie* dish into the hospital. Everyone has his or her own idea of boundaries and of insecurities, and this just didn't strike me as being very manly. Being a nurse definitely made me sensitive about protecting and defending my masculinity. In fact, I've always hated the terms *male nurse* and *female doctor*. Why should there be such a distinction? Does one refer to *male certified public accountants* or *female lawyers*?

In the aftermath of the Oklahoma City bombing in 1995, there was confusion about who in the emergency room was in charge because everyone wore the same color scrubs. Taking that lesson to heart, I began to wear a white lab coat to distinguish myself as the charge nurse in ICU and make it easier for doctors who needed to find me quickly. New Doctor Resident Jasmine was especially attentive to me. She treated me like a king. Later, I discovered my lapel was covering my name tag, and I moved it so that it could be seen. The resident approached me, looked at my name tag, and said, "Oh, you're just a nurse." Because I was wearing white and was a male, she had assumed I was a doctor. I was "just" a nurse.

Despite my insecurities, I would do almost anything for my fellow nurses, and besides, not many other people ever walked the eight flights of the back stairway. Occasionally, I would meet busy Doctor C going up with a "five-flight lunch" in hand, but he would be too engrossed in finishing his meal before reaching the fifth floor to notice what I might be carrying. From the stairway, it would be a quick walk down a short hallway to the ICU with Tracey's lunch.

"Sure, Tracey. What does it look like?"

"It's on the bottom shelf of the refrigerator, and it's in a Victoria's Secret bag."

"I'm sorry, Tracey. I can't do that. I don't have the self-esteem to carry a Victoria's Secret bag throughout the hospital. What if someone saw me carrying that bag? You'll have to find someone else."

Later that day, an eighteen-year-old boy involved in a motor vehicle crash was admitted to the ICU with non-life-threatening injuries. I assigned Nurse Don to be his *primary* nurse, which meant that whenever Don worked, he would be this young man's nurse. Don and I had been friends for many years, and I had in fact been an usher at his wedding a few months prior. He married Samantha, an X-ray technician at the same hospital where we worked, and both were regarded as highly respected, skilled caregivers.

On the second morning with this patient, Don took report on the teen, gave the 8:00 am medications, and went out to talk with the family and tell them what was being planned for the day.

"I need to give him a bath," he began. "I should be done in about thirty minutes. The cafeteria is open, if you'd like to go there during this time. When I'm done, you'll be able to see him again."

Things do not always go as planned in nursing, as interruptions are common. Before Don could give the young man his bath, the primary physician wanted to make rounds and spent twenty minutes with Don's patient. The physician wrote out an assortment of orders, including an electrocardiogram (EKG) and an arterial blood gas. When Don was completing oversight of these tests 15 minutes later, the consulting orthopedic surgeon walked in and spent thirty minutes with them. By that time, Don needed to give the next hour's medications, suction and institute a tube feeding with his other patient, and chart the morning's progress.

By the time three hours had elapsed, Don still wasn't done with the bath. I saw the family come to the door several times during this interlude and told them Don was not yet finished with their son's bath due to other pressing needs.

Nurse Karen G heard me muttering under my breath about the family's impatience and patted me on the back. "That's all they can see, Ray. It's not their fault." She was right, and I nodded in agreement.

Secretary Pam prided herself in always being on top of family dynamics. She possessed an uncanny ability, in fact, to appear busy in an empty room. During the week prior, two ministers, under the protective eyes of the law, had visited with patients' families. According to the *Bangor Daily News*, one was accused of pounding his organist. Parishioners beat the other minister with chains after he'd taken a minor into the church for "deprogramming" without the parents' permission. Pam had quipped that they should get together and start a new church called "Dick 'Em and Deck 'Em." Now she was telling me that the family of Don's patient wanted to speak to the person in charge.

Past experience and observation of other nurses have taught me about families. A family typically speaks to the nurse in charge to voice complaints, not compliments. The majority of families don't appreciate that a nurse may have listened to a patient's lungs and, having assessed they are full of fluid, may have determined the patient needs a diuretic. Nor do they see that a nurse may be regulating and adjusting a powerful medication being dripped to control a patient's blood pressure, or that a nurse may be assessing a wound that has become infected. A family sees only what its eyes can see, and a caregiver should avoid extricating a family from the situation. As Dr. D liked to say, "The patient or family waiting for you is counting your faults." Once I accepted this, I became a better nurse in the eyes of the family, and I took the time, for example, to trim the hair out of the ears and nostrils of older men who came into our unit. If their eyebrows were long and overhanging, I would trim those too.

As was my practice, I went first to the nurse to ask him if he knew what the family might want to speak to me about. Satisfied I knew the nurse's position, I approached the family.

"We'd like you to take the male nurse off our son's case," they said to me. "He seems a little 'too nice,' if you know what I mean."

"I'm afraid I don't. Don is one of our best nurses---"

"You know, *homo-sexual*," the father enunciated, holding up a limp wrist. Obviously a religious man, the father then launched into a three-minute sermon about the "evils" of homosexuality.

Don is a very manly man. I could only surmise they were suspicious due to the length of time it had taken to give the bath. Personally, even if Don were gay, I knew homosexuality and professionalism are in no way mutually exclusive. I looked at our tight staffing and evaluated who might best be able to soften the family dynamics in this case without negatively impacting the care of an already-assigned patient or family. With a little ripple of self-satisfaction, I assigned the only person I could spare to take Don's place and satisfy the family.

When I broke the news to Don, he was very upset, and he seemed confused about the amusement written across my face. The whole situation was absurd, and I couldn't keep a straight face, despite sensing that his self-esteem had taken a nosedive. But when I told Don whom I'd assigned to take his place, he joined me in a satisfied little laugh. I had replaced him with the best person available: an all-American, young, pretty, hard-working, conscientious, engaging, witty, Southern Baptist, Bible-thumping . . . lesbian.

"Difficult times have helped me to understand better than before, how infinitely rich and beautiful life is in every way, and that so many things that one goes worrying about are of no importance whatsoever." ~Isak Dinesen, author

No two families are exactly alike, and we do well to remember the importance of being present in a way that is meaningful to each. Sometimes families make requests which at first sound absurd but in reality make a lot of sense. Such was the case with Fred and Anna.

Fred was a diabetic most of his adult life but rarely saw a physician. People have lots of excuses for avoiding doctors. Commonly, people feel that they are sicker after seeing a doctor than before or that they get loaded up with too many medications. It seems that, in their minds, unless an illness is validated in some way, it doesn't exist and has no power over them.

Fred had injured his foot while working in the woods of northern Maine, and gangrene had set in. Gangrene can spread to other parts of the body, which would be fatal, and the recourse in such cases is amputation of the affected body part before the gangrene can spread. But in Fred's case, due to advanced metastatic cancer with bowel obstruction, death within a few weeks was a certainty even without the gangrenous complication.

Anna was very proud that her husband had been a hardworking man all of his life. She accepted his imminent death, but she was apprehensive about cutting off his foot, especially since the justification was to "prevent premature death" in someone who would die soon anyway. Because Fred was not conscious, she made the difficult decision to leave the foot intact. A tourniquet was applied around the line of demarcation (which separates affected from unaffected tissue), and the foot was placed in a plastic bag filled with dry ice. We call this *physiological amputation*. In this way, Fred's body was preserved intact for his burial.

Candlelight illuminated the faces of a couple in their seventies. She was a pretty lady with silver gray hair in soft curls surrounding a round face with velveteen, rosy cheeks and sparkling blue eyes. As she peered at the menu, the little pearls of a golden chain holding her glasses around her neck dangled playfully back and forth in the glow of the flickering light. She smiled radiantly at the man sitting to her left. He was much taller, and his hair was white, as white as the snow that lay out beyond the window of this little café. One could drown in the depth of his dark brown eyes, which were overshadowed by bushy white eyebrows.

"How about the salmon?" she asked. "They have the sauce you are so fond of."

Her companion was examining the fine details of the cream-colored lace tablecloth and for a moment was lost in its intricacy. The pattern reminded him of something he'd seen before, something fancy and precious.

"Earl," she continued. The waiter looked at the lady and then at the gentleman and then quickly back at the lady. "Bring us each a toasted almond. And we'll have the poached salmon, baked potato, and asparagus almondine."

They sat sipping their cocktails for a good hour, staring at each other with gentle smiles and occasionally interjecting comments about the crackling log fire, the soft music, or the couples who sat near their table. Secretly, the gentleman stole glances at this sweet lady while she wasn't looking and marveled that such a pretty lady would have accompanied him there. When dinner came, they savored every tender, juicy morsel and laughed heartily when the gentleman dropped butter in his water glass.

"They'll be wondering what was wrong with the water they were serving when they see this in the dish room," she said, chuckling and winking at the man.

All in all, it was a wonderful evening, and the aromas lingered just a bit, as if they were soaking up all the memories. At last, the man spoke to this lovely lady. "I like you," he said shyly. "Do you think you might want to see me or go out with me again sometime?" he asked hesitantly, his voice steeped in trepidation and his eyes colored with hope.

"It would be my honor," she answered, tears welling up in her eyes. She counted out some crisp dollar bills and laid them on the table next to the glass of yellow, greasy water. Then she helped him up from his chair, extinguished the candlelight, put on her coat, and walked her husband back to the home they had shared for the last fifty years.

Alzheimer's disease has been described as death by a thousand subtractions. Dr. Phil Peverada shared the story above with me as a poignant reminder that the patient's caregiver deserves our compassion and attention too. In this story, Earl's wife met the adversity of a devastating disease with grace and compassion. She accepted the challenge by choosing to look at it not as a burden, but as a privilege and honor in serving someone she loves: a final, parting gift.

". . . For you will still be here tomorrow, but your dreams may not."
~Cat Stevens, singer

Just as the caregiver of the Alzheimer patient in the previous scenario may be a family member, nurses are sometimes present when one of their own family members dies. It is important to remember roles are reversed in such situations, and caregivers are grieving, in need of the same compassion they extend to relative strangers at other times. Words do not have to pass in order for caring to be communicated.

Such was the case when on one Easter Sunday morning Larry was admitted to the ICU after sustaining a ruptured cerebral aneurysm. Larry was a handsome man of thirty-six and the father of two small children. Accompanying him was his wife Ruth Ellen, who was the sister of ICU's Nurse Julie.

Within a few hours of arriving at the medical center, Larry was taken to the OR for a clipping of the aneurysm. Surgery to repair it went well, but postoperatively Larry's brain began to swell, his condition deteriorated, and we began to prepare for the inevitable. When my shift ended on the evening of Larry's tenth day with us, I put on my jacket and bid a gentle goodnight to Ruth Ellen, who sat and kept vigil with Larry in his darkened room.

What happened next was something Ruth Ellen will never forget. She writes,

> The night before Larry was pronounced "brain dead," I was in his darkened room alone and had what I believe to be the amazing experience of witnessing Larry's spirit leaving his body. There was a moment when it appeared someone was adjusting a dimmer switch with . . . some degree of unearthly . . . light going up, then down. [It was] . . . not like an electrical surge, but as if there was a switch that could be

138

turned up and down slightly. Not poetic enough to give the right illusion that I witnessed. Whatever it was, it was my message from Larry that he was gently leaving a body that was no longer useful to him and that he was heading to someplace more serene. It was quite peaceful, serene . . . [and] it truly gave me an inner peace.

When Julie came into the room a few minutes later, I asked if she or another staff member had adjusted the lights earlier, and she said, "Ruth, the light switches are at the head of the bed." The door was near the foot of the bed.

Later, she would write,

> [The experience in Larry's room that night] gave, and has continued to give me, such peace with Larry's passing. You [Ray] had a lot to do with this by recognizing the importance of keeping patient environments peaceful and serene. You invited that experience to be welcomed and to be witnessed, and I will remember it for the rest of my life. Thank you so very much for all you did for Larry. That experience and your loving care helped lessen the unpleasant memories of that time in the lives of my children and myself.

Dr. S pronounced Larry brain dead the following evening and made the decision to keep Larry on a ventilator so that the family could visit the next morning. He also did not want Larry to be discontinued from mechanical support late at night, after which the family might arrive home in the wee hours of the morning without the support of other family members.

"Ray, could you please see that Larry's fingernails are trimmed?" Ruth Ellen simply asked before she left.

As was my usual practice after a death, I set about the ministry of involving myself with the family. Because one of our own had sustained this loss, the case had a pronounced effect on the entire medical staff. We were saddened and aware of Ruth Ellen's heavy burden. Not only did she have to deal with the loss of her "Sweet" Larry, but she also had to assist her two young children in accepting his death, and she had to keep daily activities going. The couple had owned and operated a variety store near our medical center, and she had to continue to keep it running. The neurosurgeon was so moved by our sadness that he later gifted each of the ICU staff two tickets to a local movie theater.

The next morning, Ruth Ellen laughed when she noticed how short I'd cut Larry's fingernails. Then she looked around the room in amazement. The radio was set to a station playing soft music; the blinds were closed, and the lights were dimmed. Looking back at Larry, she noticed his hands were placed on top of the covers for those who might want to hold his hand, the bed rails were lowered on both sides of the bed, and chairs and boxes of tissues were placed on each side of the bed. She turned and smiled at me approvingly.

"I wanted it to be welcoming to family members who might want to say any last words," I explained.

One of our other nurses breezed by on her way to retrieve something, and she commented, "It looks like a funeral parlor in here! It's perfect."

"Thank you," I said, happy to have achieved my goal.

After the family's visit with their departed loved one, Nurse Julie hugged each as they left. She turned to me and said, "I saved the best hug for you!"

As nurses, we must be ready to lend support to families of patients who have died or who are expected to die. While acknowledging emotional baggage derived from our own similar circumstances, we must summon a great deal of strength to help us remain in control and focused on others. As Dr. L liked to say, we need to "maintain a therapeutic relationship one hundred percent of the time."

Nurse Myrna was a mother of three boys when she came to work in the ICU, and like many of us, she found it particularly difficult when dealing with the loss of young people. We are indebted to her for sharing the following three encounters.

Like many young married couples in their early thirties, Libby and Greg were expecting. This would be, in fact, their second child, and though the pregnancy was a surprise, the couple and their seven-year-old daughter were looking forward to and preparing for the blessed event.

A newspaper delivery employee, Libby would usually walk several miles a day on her route, but in her seventeenth week of pregnancy Libby was not feeling well. She blamed it initially on the pregnancy but resorted to being seen in the emergency room when things continued to seem amiss. There she was diagnosed with a urinary tract infection, prescribed an antibiotic, and sent home. Later she was admitted to the ICU in septic shock, which progressed to acute respiratory distress syndrome. The privilege of being Libby's primary nurse fell to Nurse Myrna, who spoke briefly with Libby before Libby became so ill that she needed to be heavily sedated and placed on full mechanical support.

"Will my baby be okay?" she asked.

"We'll do everything we can for you and your baby. Right now, you're having trouble breathing. We can breathe better for you with this machine than you can do on your own. And we have to give you some stuff to make you sleep so you don't remember this tube in your throat

141

and you don't feel any pain with it. You're also not going to be able to talk because the tube will be in your voice box. Why don't you spend a few minutes with your husband and little girl before we do that?"

Having a patient on mechanical support is almost always harder on the family than on the patient. Family members find the tubes and machines and noises foreign, obtrusive, and scary, while the patient is unaware. Because her condition was deteriorating rapidly, there was little time for much exchange except the usual "I love you," hugs and kisses.

Libby's husband, Greg, was exceptionally kind and patient. He came every morning after seeing little Kara onto the school bus and stayed by Libby's side until it was time for Kara to come home. Sometimes he would bring Kara in to see "Mommy" after supper, as Kara was accustomed to family time before going to bed. She would kiss Libby's face and wish her "sweet dreams" when Greg finished reading to them all.

On her sixth day in the unit, Libby took a turn for the worse. Her blood pressure dropped dramatically, and doctors feared her organs would soon begin to fail. As a last-ditch measure to relieve the stress on her body and preserve her life, an abortion was considered. It fell to Myrna, who had come to know the family well, to help Greg work through all the aspects of the difficult question posed by her physician.

"Greg," she gently began, "Libby's life is slipping away. Doctors feel she might have a better chance if she doesn't also have to fight for the baby's life."

Greg didn't want to have to make that decision. He walked slowly toward the door, shaking his head.

"I can't," he finally said. "I can't."

Myrna put her hand on Greg's shoulder and then left the two of them alone for the remainder of the afternoon. The doctor had taken measures to bring Libby's blood pressure back up temporarily, and she would not require an answer before the following morning. Greg would surely need some time to come to terms with this. Greg and Libby had always made tough decisions together. He recalled their decision just a few months earlier to buy their new home. With the new baby coming, they'd both felt it was important to provide more space. Now they faced a much tougher decision. He made arrangements for Kara to go to his sister's house that evening, and he stayed to "talk to" Libby.

Myrna thought of her own young family and made sure Greg knew he could confide in her and could count on her being a willing listener. But Greg knew Libby was the only person who could help him with this. She was his partner---"for better or for worse"---and it couldn't get much "worse" than this.

He was still by her bedside when Myrna came in the following morning. His tear-stained face stared up at her when she entered Libby's room.

"I want Libby to live," he said. "Do whatever it takes."

Myrna choked back her own tears and nodded. As the bedside abortion got underway, Myrna felt strongly that this poor woman would not survive. A few days later, with Greg by her side, Libby went into respiratory and cardiac arrest. Efforts to revive her were unsuccessful. Greg was still there with Libby as Myrna disconnected the tubes and wires and cleaned her lifeless body.

"Libby," he said. "There's a huge hole in my heart. How can I go on without you?"

Libby's physician sat down beside him.

"Eight years ago, I had a baby boy," she began. "He was the joy of my life, so beautiful, always smiling and happy. He was just starting to say words like 'da da' and 'ma ma,' when we lost him. He was gone so suddenly that it didn't seem as if it could possibly be true. We put him to bed, and one moment he was sleeping peacefully, the next he was gone. They said it was sudden infant death syndrome. My life seemed like a jigsaw puzzle on a table that had been turned upside down. All of the puzzle pieces were scattered and no longer fit neatly together with the other pieces. It took a long, long time to put the puzzle back together again . . . One piece will always be missing. Losing someone you love is like that . . . I'm so sorry."

Libby's doctor and Myrna sat with Greg for almost an hour as he held his wife's hand and cried. The doctor's caring words had helped him to begin the long process of grief, which must end with acceptance.

"And when my heart's dearest died, the light went out from my life forever."
~Theodore Roosevelt on his wife's death

"Profound loss, heartache, and despair are as much a part of life as happiness and joy."
~Becky Pelletier, Fayette, Maine

For many, Christmas is a joyous occasion marked by memories of happy family gatherings. For others who are separated from loved ones, especially when the holiday marks a tragic anniversary, its joy can accentuate and magnify feelings of loneliness or loss. When Nurse Myrna offered to cover the evening shift three days prior to Christmas of 1980, little did she know the holiday would usher in tragic circumstances in the ICU for the families of three local teens.

Two adolescent boys and one adolescent girl were dead, facts that seemed to justify Myrna's contention that it was a "crapshoot" whether or not a teen can make it to adulthood. A vehicle had struck one of the boys as he was walking in the darkness of the previous night. He had been a nursing student, home on Christmas break. The other boy was a young driver involved in a motor vehicle crash blamed on snowy conditions. The boys were declared brain dead, and we were awaiting recovery of organs donated by the grieving parents.

The third victim was Myrna's patient. She was a college student, who had been out rushing around doing last-minute Christmas shopping.

"Make sure you drive slowly---the roads are icy," her mother had warned.

She was known as a careful driver and never needed reminding about wearing her seat belt.

"Don't worry," she'd said. "I won't be gone long."

In what should have only been a fender-bender, her car was hit from behind while she was going a conservative 30 miles per hour. The impact caused her to jolt forward and lose consciousness, and it is believed that prolonged contact with the seat belt against her neck while awaiting ambulance transport resulted in a clot, which traveled to her brain.

Lying in the hospital bed, she looked completely untouched. She did not resemble the typical patients who come to the ICU after motor vehicle crashes. Such patients often are close to being unrecognizable, covered in lacerations and bruises, and attached to all manner of wires and tubes (giving the unit a reputation for being an almost intolerable experience). But this girl looked as if she were simply asleep.

"Is she going to be O.K.?" the mother asked the physician as he escorted her and her husband and two younger siblings into the room where the girl lay.

"I'm afraid she has died," he said. As he rambled on in sympathy and explanation, the remaining words were lost in oblivion as the family struggled to come to terms with the fact that she was dead.

Their shocked silence came to life suddenly when the girl's brother launched into a rage and began with heaving sobs to punch the wall. As the charge nurse worked to calm the girl's brother, the rest of the family hung their heads in overwhelming grief and sorrow. Myrna felt her heart would surely burst. Though Myrna was an exceptionally empathetic person with the ability to communicate what was needed at the right time, she felt horribly inadequate and unable to explain or help in such circumstances. She felt faint and later took her temperature. It was three degrees higher than normal. She wished she could have been home to hug her three boys.

When Myrna returned for duty the next day, the girl had already left the unit for organ recovery. She felt comforted there were other families somewhere in the world whose children would receive a gift of life on this Christmas Day.

"You can celebrate what you can still do or mourn what you lost."
~Author Unknown

It took just seconds to make the decision. Flames licked the threshold of the small garage apartment, and black smoke began to close in on where they stood in their nightclothes. There was only one way out.

"Jump!" he cried. "It's only twenty feet. I'll go first, and you'll see—promise me you'll follow!"

With reassurance from her, he jumped to the ground below. Despite a broken ankle, Robert immediately stood up and held out his arms to encourage his wife. Grace looked at the flames, turned back to Robert, and made a desperate leap. It would forever change her life.

Twenty-seven-year-old Grace was eight months pregnant, which altered her center of balance and caused her to fall backward, breaking her neck. She was rendered a quadriplegic, able to move her head and neck but unable to effect more than spastic movements from her arms down to her feet. Her blood pressure also dropped, decreasing the blood supply to her baby and leading to the baby's demise. During surgery, she bled and required a hysterectomy. Later she was told she could never have any children of her own. She ended up on a ventilator due to an inability to maintain her respiratory status.

Robert felt totally helpless. When his infant daughter was brought from the morgue, he was at least able to hold her for a short time, something Grace could not do. Nurse Myrna laid the baby next to Grace so that she could at least see her. The baby looked perfect, as if she were only sleeping.

"She's beautiful," Grace mouthed, tears in her eyes.

Day after day, Grace would lie in her bed and cry, thinking about all of the things in life taken from her and her family. She would never walk again. She could never be the kind of wife to Robert she wanted to be, could never hold him in her arms. She'd lost the only biological child she would ever have. She'd lost her home and all her worldly possessions.

Despite her overwhelming feelings of pity for this woman, Myrna did not project her own fears. Myrna reminded her what a devoted and loving husband she had. She told Grace how very much Robert needed her, especially now. Myrna told her how very much Robert needed to be needed and loved by *her.* Grace and her husband slowly adjusted, until at last she was able to go to a new home, a home Robert built with handicapped-accessible ramps, lots of windows, and no second floor.

"The Lord is near to the broken hearted and saves those who are crushed in spirit."
~Psalms 34: Verse 18

Subchapter 2: Acceptance

Though we are unique as individuals, there are certain spiritual needs common to all of us. We all have an intrinsic need for love of an unconditional nature, a love that will survive anything, even destruction of our physical bodies. This is the undying and dedicated love of a mother for a child born with multiple challenges, for example. The underlying issue is that people be loved for who, not what, they are. We also have a need for meaning and purpose in life. What difference did it make in the world that we were ever born? As we saw in the story about Jack in Part 1 of "Loss," the need for forgiveness is also universal, as humans do not deal very effectively with guilt over long periods of time.

Similarly, the human need for hope must also be nourished. If there is hope for a cure, a patient can hope for the things life after illness can bring: walking a daughter down the matrimonial aisle, ice cream in the park, celebrating next year's birthday with a spouse. Nurse Dean, as he sometimes did on his days off, took a group of quadriplegics to a pool for swimming therapy. Most of the group were already in the pool when Billy, who had recently begun to regain a little mobility after months in a wheelchair, hobbled red-faced toward the pool using a walker. His jerky, unsteady gait validated the effort it must have taken for each painful step, and his comrades in the pool watched him in awe.

"F*** you, Billy!" one of his companions yelled out. "Stop walking!"

These men formed a cohesive group because of their shared disability and because of their shared *acceptance* of each other's disability and hope for improvements. Acceptance allowed them to still enjoy life and even encourage one in their group with a bit of humor.

Healing without cure involves redirecting one's hope toward more immediate concerns: a walk in the sunshine, resolution of unresolved conflicts, emotional well-being, a pain-free death, or even Heaven. Why should terminally ill patients or their families be stripped of feeling any measure of hope? Spiritual needs such as these often cannot begin to be addressed before there is some degree of acceptance: acceptance of an imperfection, acceptance of not having achieved fame, acceptance that allows one to let go of anger, and acceptance of the impermanence of life.

Many years and experiences into nursing, I was involved in trying to console the mother of a teenage boy who was dying from a self-inflicted gunshot wound. He was a tall young man, whose buff body took up the full length of the bed. His short-cropped black hair and tan, muscular upper body boldly contradicted the occasion and begged the question of how someone who'd taken such good care of himself physically had veered so off course emotionally. This was a snapshot at the end of what I knew was a much bigger picture of conflict for both of them.

"We may never know what drove your son to do this."

She took another Kleenex from the brightly colored box in her limp hands and covered her eyes. I looked at the stringy, blonde hair hanging in her worry-lined face and noticed the gray starting to show at her temples. What thoughts were going through her tormented mind at such a time? She had been both a mother and a father to her boy. Was his whole life flashing before her: changing his diapers, hearing his first words, seeing him ride his bike for the first time, hugging him when he brought in to her a clump of sod covered with bluets the first Mother's Day he was aware of the occasion—the best he could have managed without a father's help? Did she wonder if a father in his life would have made a difference? Frequently, parents harbor a sense of guilt for their children's actions.

"Who knows? There might even have been an organic anomaly such as a brain lesion. You did the best you could do," I added.

We were sustaining the boy on mechanical support pending determination of brain death and request of his organs from the family, and I briefly left the mother with my peer, Nurse Madonna, while attending to another patient. As I walked out of the room, Nurse Amy called me into the next room.

"What you said to the mother was really beautiful," she said. It was moments like these, affirmation from those who share the challenges, that all nurses appreciate.

In my absence, the mother related the story of her son's triumphant winning of a trophy in a chess tournament a few years earlier. Walking into the room, unaware of the mother's story, I heard Madonna say, "He must have been tickled to death."

I looked at the patient's lifeless body in the bed and then at Madonna. She immediately picked up on my nonverbal, put her hands to her face, and said to the mother, "Oh, I'm so sorry I said that."

The mother, on the other hand, upon seeing my expression, broke out into a cathartic laugh, hesitant at first, and then growing into a tear-filled, full belly laugh. It was not long after that the mom was able to accept her son's brain death and consent to gift his organs.

There is a calmness that acceptance of our mortality bestows. Instead of fearing the inevitable, we are freed to celebrate what life has to offer each day that we awaken. Hope and faith are wonderful vessels, but acceptance gives us freedom to live each day to the fullest, taking nothing for granted, and giving fully of ourselves.

With long, flowing golden locks, a creamy, soft complexion, sparkling green eyes, and a bright smile, Jessica was a beauty, and she was encouraged at an early age to enter beauty pageants. Her six-foot, 125-pound frame was stunning. She was the apple of her father's eye, and he showed her off to his friends and coworkers every opportunity he got. If he was scheduled to show a house to a client after her high school let out for the day, he would ask her to accompany them. If he needed to hold an open house, he would ask Jessica to show the prospective buyers around. It was also a way for Jessica to earn a little money, which she eagerly put toward her college fund.

"Jess," he called one day. "Could you show a house today after classes?"

"Sure thing, Dad. Where's the house?"

As her father relayed the address, he thought what an impression she would make with the prospective buyers and added, "The prospectus and key will be in the lockbox on the front door. You have the code. They should be there by 3:30, and I'll be along around 3:45. Thanks, Sweetie."

Jessica closed her cell phone and tucked it back into her backpack, noticing her lunchtime was almost over. Besides her outward beauty, she was a stellar student and got along well with everyone. She didn't really mind helping her father. She just wished he might take notice at some point of her own interests. Had he forgotten her piano recital was that evening?

At 2:50 Jessica hurried to her locker and picked up the few things she would need to take home. She hastened to the parking lot, resisting the temptation to chat with some of her friends along the way. Turning the key in the ignition, she glanced again at the address her father had given her before backing out of her space and pulling out onto Route 1A.

When Jessica's father arrived at the appointed time, he was surprised to see his clients still waiting in their car and Jessica's car nowhere in sight. He hit speed dial as he walked toward his clients. There was no answer.

"I'm terribly sorry to keep you waiting," he said to his clients. "My daughter is usually right on time."

By the time he finished showing the house, his cell phone rang. It was his wife.

"Jess is in the hospital. There's been a car accident."

The trip from the house to the hospital was a total blur, and he quickly found himself walking toward a huddle of physicians and family members. Seeing him, they parted to let him in.

"How is she?" he asked.

A physician in green surgical scrubs looked up. "We're taking her into surgery now. She's sustained a severe head injury, and we need to evacuate a cerebral hematoma. I'm afraid this is a very serious injury."

Jessica had suffered the misfortune of crashing into a moose on I-395. Though she lived, she'd lost the ability to function in any kind of meaningful way. During her stay in the ICU, she never opened her eyes or interacted with anyone. Except for the first day, I never saw the father come in.

"Where is your husband?" I asked his wife one day. "Is he unable to come in?" While we may try our best to be objective and to not pass judgment, we are, after all, human and imperfect. As a group committed to caring for this teen, we began to chatter amongst ourselves and to question why the father hadn't taken the time to come in and see his daughter. The chief executive of a large company, could the man not make a few minutes to show his unconditional love? Oftentimes, there are extenuating circumstances to which we are not privy and which explain why a loved one may not be present as expected, and I hoped to put the chatter to rest once and for all. Phrasing the question delicately was crucial.

Jessica's mother told me her husband could not bear looking at his once beautiful daughter, who had been reduced in his mind to a mass of tissue. He was so broken up by what had happened to her that he could not physically bring himself to come into the unit.

"It is only with the heart that one can see rightly; what is essential is invisible to the eye."
~Antoine De Saint-Exupéry, *The Little Prince*

"Sometimes it is the artist's task to find out how much music you can still make with what you have left."
~Itzhak Perlman, violinist

As ICU nurses who have cared for many patients, we often receive cards and letters expressing patients' gratitude for our care in bringing them back from the edge of death. One such card stood out from the others because it was written in a most elegant and exquisite calligraphy. The bright, bold lettering was written on stationery flooded with the vivid colors of a hand-painted Maine seascape.

"Dear Nurses," it began. "I am writing this with a pen between my lips. You may remember me. I came into the ICU two years ago with a high, complete spinal cord transection." She went on to explain how she'd discovered the unique talent of writing, drawing, and painting with her lips. I glanced down at the signature before continuing. "Serenity," it was signed.

How could we forget Serenity? She was a lovely, slender girl just shy of her eighteenth birthday in the summer of 1984, and she had the misfortune of having been involved in a motor vehicle crash that left her an instant quadriplegic. Her prognosis included the promise of no more than gross motor movement in her upper extremities and no movement at all in her legs. Because of the complete cord transection, there was no room for anything more hopeful. The nurses were not accustomed to seeing a female in this condition, as most quadriplegics are male due to their greater tendency for high-risk behaviors.

Within a very short time after her admission, we were able to tell her with almost one hundred percent certainty she would never be able to walk again. She was at the point at which her lungs were becoming fatigued and her cough was becoming weaker. In a couple of days, she would need to be intubated to help her breathe. By that time, she would reach the age of majority in the state of Maine---considered capable of making her own decisions at the age of eighteen---and she made it clear that did not want to live like this. Serenity did not want either heroic actions or life-sustaining measures, such as a ventilator, to keep her alive. She wanted nature to take its course. Half of the nursing staff agreed with her, and the other half disagreed. How could someone so young and in such a state of shock, disbelief, and fear be competent to make such a life-changing decision?

Her parents were also split about this decision. To this day, I think of how unselfish one parent was—how much love it took---to be willing to accept the daughter's decision to die. I was equally impressed with the other parent, who could see a strength in the daughter that the parent believed would deliver her from despair in the end.

The dilemma we as medical professionals are constantly facing is that it is much harder to remove life-saving measures than it is to institute them. Once patients are on dialysis, it's hard to discontinue it. Once they are intubated, it's much harder to take them off the ventilator prematurely. There was a similar case prior to this in which a young man had come in with a stroke from a cerebral aneurysm. In that case, almost all of the nursing staff and primary and consulting physicians felt and told the family there was no hope of his ever escaping a persistent vegetative state. In front of the families, I usually support decisions made by the medical staff. But in this case, I didn't, for I had seen movements in the patient indicative of a better response than what they were predicting. I was so bold as to even have stated one day to the father, "I think your son is going to walk out of here." A year later, the boy and his father walked into our waiting room. The father told me the lad was helping him in his grocery store in Winter Harbor and appreciated my being the only one who'd shared a positive attitude about his son, the only one who'd given him any hope. Though I was happy about the outcome, it was something I never did again, for making such bold predictions has an equal chance of backfiring and giving false hope to those already in delicate circumstances. All my experiences now made me pause, where once I had felt so certain.

We debated the merits of each side of Serenity's case for weeks until, in the end, we as a group of physicians, nurses, other medical professionals, and family decided to keep her going. Once most patients pass through our doors, we never see or hear from them again. Serenity's letter was a poignant reminder that decisions made in part by the medical staff can be life-changing.

I continued reading, hoping to find some hint of closure regarding our decision. The words seemed to jump right off the page and caress my face.

"Thank you," it read. "I'm so happy to be alive!"

Life is an opportunity, benefit from it.
Life is beauty, admire it. Life is bliss, taste it.
Life is a dream, realize it. Life is a challenge, meet it.
Life is a duty, complete it. Life is a game, play it.
Life is a promise, fulfill it. Life is sorrow, overcome it.
Life is a song, sing it. Life is a struggle, accept it.
Life is a tragedy, confront it. Life is an adventure, dare it.
Life is luck, make it.
Life is too precious, do not destroy it.
Life is life, fight for it.
~Mother Teresa

"Life is like an onion: You peel it off one layer at a time, and sometimes you weep."
~ Carl Sandburg, poet

One afternoon in late winter, I was assigned to care for an 84-year-old woman who reminded me of my own mother. My mother had passed away just a few months earlier. Like my mother, Elsie was gentle, quiet, and patient. In contrast to my mother, who was surrounded by all twelve of her children on her deathbed, Elsie was alone.

As she lay dying in her bed, she told me she was afraid of death. As she spoke of her years working as an artist, I followed the outline of the veins in her long, thin fingers to the spot in her arm where I had inserted her IV. Her arms were gaunt and pale. *How could they have possibly shaped clay or held a paintbrush?* I wondered.

As she spoke in a heavy French-Canadian accent of the loneliness of recent years, I began to regard her personhood as a precious jewel.

Every white hair, every wrinkle etched from time and experience, every imperfection became witness to the sacrifices and the challenges life had thrown her way. In talking with Elsie, I noticed she never pronounced the letter *H*, undoubtedly a carryover from her native language French, in which the *H* is also silent.

"Dere are good tings and bad tings about growing old," she confided.

"Tell me about that."

"Da good ting is obviously dat you can live a long time and enjoy da good tings of dis Eart. Old age is a privilege dat not everyone enjoys."

"And the bad? I asked.

"Well, da bad is dat you experience tings you'd radder not. My only child died before me, and I lost my 'usband before dat—some tirty years ago now. In fact, I wrote a poem about my son after 'e died. 'E was only sixteen years old."

Her voice got weaker, and I leaned closer to her head to hear her whispers. She proceeded to recite the poem.

"Memories dat fall like petals from da pages of my mind . . ."

As I held her hand, she finished reciting, and I proceeded to ask her about everything else I could think of that would be important for her to relay. Where did she grow up? What was her son like? What kinds of art did she excel at? I wanted to know everything.

"Just before my son turned fourteen, I tought I would teach 'im how to drive. Where I grew up, dat's da way my parents 'ad taught me. Anyway, I sat in da passenger seat and 'e sat be'ind da steering wheel, and we started to roll down Main Street in Brewer. A policeman saw us and turned on 'is siren. My son pulled da car over like 'e'd been doing it all 'is life."

"What did you tell the policeman?"

"I told 'im I was teaching my son 'ow to drive, and da policeman looked at me like I 'ad t'ree heads. 'E's a little young, isn't 'e, Ma'am?' 'e asked me. Den 'e asked me if 'e 'ad a license, to which I replied dat 'e certainly did not—'E's only tirteen and a 'alf.'"

"Then what?"

"The policeman den just told me dat we couldn't do dat and dat I 'ad to drive da car. So, we switched positions and I drove da car home. In fact, I drove it for da next t'irty years—even dough I never 'ad a driver's license myself."

Elsie had grown up in Eagle Lake, Maine, a northern Maine town of about eight hundred residents, mostly Francophones. The daughter of a lumberjack, she'd known a life of poverty until meeting her husband, and they had carved out a life for themselves and their child farther south in Penobscot County. While he supported the family as an electrician for a local hospital, her aspirations to become an artist were realized, and she had opened a little shop to sell her paintings. These, she told me, were mostly landscapes done in watercolors, the brighter the better.

"Looking at drabness only makes you feel drab," she said.

Because I was the charge nurse for the unit that day, I was responsible for attending patients who needed emergency resuscitations, which we called *codes*. As luck would have it, a code was called a few doors down the hall, and I found myself in the difficult situation of leaving this lovely woman by herself. Instinctively, I leaned over the remaining few inches to her forehead and kissed her gently. "I have to go," I said, "but I'll be back."

The kiss might be frowned upon by most today, but it was a natural, uncomplicated response to a difficult circumstance and the best thing I could have done with so little time. An infant first experiences love through touch, and we never outgrow the need. Not all patients, of course, like to be touched, but I knew this would be meaningful and reassuring for Elsie. After forty-five minutes at the code, I returned to

Elsie's bedside, foregoing my lunch and anxious to learn more of her story.

"I'm back," I said. "Sorry I was gone so long, but it was one of . . ."

My words trailed off, as I realized Elsie was not listening. Her eyes had closed one last time. Her lips would forever be still. While I was succeeding in shocking a stranger back to life a few doors down, my friend had been quietly slipping away by herself, as unobtrusively it seemed to me as a butterfly might land on a flower petal. I again thought of my mother, whose calmness at her own death taught me people die in the same manner as they live their lives.

I had failed her, and my heart was broken. An overwhelming sadness enveloped me, shouting at me how dreadful it was that Elsie had died alone. The only peace I felt was that I'd been the last person on Earth to have held her hand or to have kissed her forehead.

Several years later on my way home from work, I happened to stop at a yard sale a few streets down from my house. The yard was strewn with piles of old books, skeins of differently colored yarns and knitting needles, crocheted afghans and homemade quilts. Walking around to the other side of these items, my eyes became fixed upon a watercolor painting framed in old gray barn board. It portrayed a green, grassy hill covered with pink and purple lupines under a bright blue sky. In the right-hand corner of the painting in petite longhand was the name "Elsie." It was if her hand had reached down from Heaven, patted me on the head, and said, "I'm doing just fine—thanks for being there."

"Life is too ironic to fully understand. It takes sadness to know what happiness is. Noise to appreciate silence. And absence to value presence."
~Author unknown

159

"For healthcare team members well versed in techniques and procedures, it is very humbling to be confronted by a patient or family member who defines meaningful support as 'just be with me.'"[12]
~Jan Pettigrew, PhD, RN

Skip was a model patient, one to whom all the nurses wanted to be assigned. He was quiet and nondemanding, he did as he was asked, and his needs were relatively simple. His good nature helped ease our load, which in the ICU can be very demanding. But silence can be a double-edged sword. Patients who have not learned trust may try to protect themselves by keeping their troubles to themselves, outwardly giving the appearance of one who is fine in every way. Inwardly, they may be one step away from disaster.

By trade Skip had been a heavy equipment operator, a job whose sometimes cold, brutal and rugged domain could be made more tolerable by a quick puff of a cigarette and a shot of brandy. Unfortunately for Skip, this would also prove to be his downfall. After twenty years of such a lifestyle, he developed a severe case of chronic obstructive pulmonary disease, commonly referred to as COPD. He was doomed to spend the rest of his days with the ICU because he needed to be on a ventilator. In those days, vented patients could not be cared for in less skilled nursing environments such as nursing homes or even in most other hospital units.

Nonetheless, Skip appeared to transition to his new world relatively unscathed. His easy, light-hearted way made him a hit with staff, who went out of their way to try and make life more tolerable for him. When the building to house the new linear accelerator was being

160

constructed between the ICU and the Grant Building, the nurses positioned Skip with his ventilator in a chair right next to the window, where he could not only watch the excavation and construction but also direct the equipment operators. The nurses would get a kick out of seeing him in his johnny at the window, waving the operators this way or the other, even halting a driver if he got too close to the building. What a good time he seemed to be having!

In his quiet demeanor, Skip always watched what the nurses were doing. Nothing escaped his eagle eyes. After eight months in the unit, he became an expert at what every switch and every monitor did and where everything was stored. If a new nurse was orienting on the unit, she'd be directed to ask Skip where the tongue blades and the gauze were kept in his room.

Skip customarily mouthed his few simple requests with one word. At Christmas, he mouthed "wine," and the nurses forwarded his request to his physician, who obliged him with a shot of red wine into his feeding tube. It was a harmless request that brought him unspeakable joy. Other times, he tried not to bother the nurses with something he felt he could handle by himself. One afternoon, Nurse Marie called me to share a precious sight. Skip had climbed up onto his bed and was squatting over his urinal in an attempt to have a bowel movement without calling for a bedpan!

It wasn't long before economics forced a change in the ICU. Management, who constantly assesses where dollars may be saved, reasoned one nurse could care for three patients like Skip, as opposed to the one-to-two nurse-to-patient ratio customary in ICU. Beds were also sometimes scarce in ICU, and Skip was occupying a bed that could have been used for a more critical patient. Why not create a step-down unit to provide a distinct environment for such patients? And so, in all the wisdom that accompanies such considerations, the new unit was created, and after eight months in ICU, Skip was transferred to the new step-down unit.

Skip now enjoyed very little access to any windows, which had connected him to the rest of the world. Besides physical suffering, he now quietly endured mental, emotional, relational, and spiritual suffering due to an isolation that left him bereft of any purpose in life. We had not yet learned to appreciate the complexity of human needs. Nor had we taken the time to ask Skip a basic question or to show him we cared. "How has the move affected how you're feeling inside? This place is quite different from where you were. I'm concerned about how you're feeling. It's important to me." These would have been lifelines for one feeling isolated, alienated, alone, and devoid of any control. These might have provided a glimmer of hope that he was not alone after all, that perhaps it was possible to make a connection or relationship in this seemingly disconnected and intimidating healthcare system he now called home. If we had only shrugged off our own disappointment at not being able to fix or cure this man's physical ills; had only resisted the temptation to turn and leave him there alone with the fancy machines. If only we had given him a *why* to live for.

But we failed. In the quiet stillness of a February night, this beautiful person disabled his vent alarm and disconnected his lifeline, allowing him to find his own way out. In his quiet, unobtrusive way, Skip made his point, and we caregivers learned a tough lesson about asking our patients the right questions and about avoiding surrogates for our therapeutic interactions. The step-down unit was closed soon after.

> To die—to sleep:
> No more; and, by a sleep to say we end
> The heart-ache and the thousand natural shocks
> That flesh is heir to, 'tis a consummation
> Devoutly to be wished. ~William Shakespeare, *Hamlet*

Acceptance derives more easily from information that is indisputable or at the very least reliable. Imagine making a decision about surgical options, if you are *lucky* enough to be the surgeon's first patient. You would likely consult another doctor before making such a life-altering decision. We would like to thank Dr. Mark S. Lingenfelter, critical care physician and pulmonologist, for sharing the following instructive experience regarding change, expertise, and acceptance.

Any new process takes time to be implemented, especially if it is a marked change from the usual routine. In 2001, a landmark paper from the University of Chicago demonstrated that "waking patients up" by stopping the sedatives they were receiving allowed them to be weaned off the ventilator significantly more quickly and to get them out of the ICU three days earlier than the usual practice standard. Additional benefits were seen with a reduction in complications, such as ventilator associated pneumonia, as well as a thirty-three percent reduction in central line infections because the patient didn't need the central line as long. Naturally, we wanted to implement the same protocol in our ICU to be sure we conformed with nationally recognized best practices. Information was disseminated through the usual channels, including physician and nurse education programs.

The abrupt cessation of sedation and analgesic medication was a marked change in ICU practice. Our nursing staff was aware of the potential for withdrawal of sedatives if they had been in place for a significant time. And abruptly shutting off sedatives was perceived as a potentially unsafe practice. (Having a patient suddenly wake up with an endotracheal tube down his throat has the potential for acute agitation with possible self-extubation or accidental central line removal.) After the plan was instituted in our ICU, it became apparent that there was a general reluctance on the part of nursing staff and perhaps even physicians.

We wanted to be sure our ICU performed at the national best practice standard but raised the question of how we could be successful at achieving our goal. Our core ICU group, consisting of multiple disciplines and managers, came to the conclusion that we would invite an outside speaker for an independent opinion regarding the implementation of the daily wake-up plan. We decided to go directly to the source and recruited Anne Pohlman, the second author of the landmark paper.

Anne was wonderful. She gave a grand rounds, in which she outlined the Chicago experience implementing the daily wake-up protocol and the outstanding results that came about after implementation. She also pointed out that they would go through cycles of being successful for a month, only to find a month later that they were implementing it only approximately fifty percent of the time, which required repeated reinforcement of its use. We wanted our nursing staff to have an opportunity to ask any question they had, and Anne went through each of our ICUs, bedside to bedside, allowing each nurse to share her questions and concerns.

Anne was such a professional. Walking down the hall and finding a piece of trash on the floor, she promptly picked it up and disposed of it before proceeding on with her goal of education in an exemplary manner.

What we immediately found after Anne's visit was nearly complete acceptance of the daily wake-up protocol. With the help of reinforcement from our core ICU group, use of the protocol achieved a more than ninety percent compliance rate. The achieved positive bedside results in turn bolstered compliance.

As I moved away from Maine to a new practice setting in different ICUs, I found that our EMMC ICU practice was far ahead in implementation of this important standard of care. At a national critical care conference in 2009, an expert in the field stated that the daily wake-up protocol was the most important study and practice implementation in the ICU in the past ten years! While the daily wake-up protocol requires coordination with extremely knowledgeable nursing staff, as well as respiratory therapists and physicians, it is extremely rewarding for patient care. I was happy to hear that when our critical care nurses went to national meetings, they found we were already doing what was being proposed as a new standard in ICU care. This had to be one of the greatest statements for an ICU medical director like me to hear, and it served as a wake-up call that getting outside assistance and expertise can make all the difference when it comes to directing change and seeking acceptance.

We as nurses are privileged to be some of the last persons some of our patients will hear, see, or touch in this world. It is an awesome responsibility. Just as we celebrate the beginning of each new life in the world, we must also be present in celebration of a life about to end. If you have ever lost someone close to you, you know how precious the memories of that person are. A person whose death is imminent also cherishes memories of his or her own life.

When my father died, the thing that impacted me most was walking into his barn after the funeral and seeing all of his tools hanging on hooks, leaning against the wall, or haphazardly left in a pile of sawdust or on a bale of hay. Everything he'd held most dear—for he was a tireless worker---was left behind. I was left to mourn the fact that he had never told me he loved me. I picked up a ratchet wrench and have it to this day, but it brings me no comfort, just a reminder that our lives and our presence with others are temporary and that if we are to enjoy the freedom of living fully, we must remember that all opportunities in life will someday be gone.

To allow dying patients this freedom means that, as much as the facts can allow, we must be gently straightforward with them about their condition. I have learned through the years not to take away *all* a family's hope, even when the situation appears hopeless. One cannot predict death one hundred per cent of the time.

I was called to attend one of our pediatric physicians, Dr R, who needed to aspirate a sample of bone marrow from a three-year-old child. The decision was made---due to complicating comorbidities—not to sedate the child. I wondered how this child would be able to handle the tremendous pain of such a procedure. Ever so gently, the physician stroked the child's hair and sang soothing words as we nurses followed suit and gently but firmly held her little arms and legs secure. Like magic, the sample was quickly obtained with little more than a whimper from the child.

I never forgot that encounter, one in which a physician---under great pressure to care for multiple patients---took the time to exert his humanity while exercising his professional skill. I felt God's presence in that room, certain that He was filling the little girl with His peace through the channels of communal care. It is this same humanity that must attend our encounters with terminally ill patients.

When we look at our patients, we must see them as our own parents, siblings, spouses, children, or friends. We must ensure we be that person unable to be present for the loved one's passing and to impart as intermediary some precious message, representing the summation of the dying person's heartfelt love, to those who arrive too

166

late. Before the Twin Towers fell, the most often relayed message from the doomed to their loved ones was a simple "I love you."

Occasionally, I encounter caregivers who through deeply personal losses of their own have found it "impossible" to return to a former position. Nurse Carina, for instance, had worked for years in the ICU, but after her father died there, she found it "impossible" to remain a nurse in the ICU and requested a transfer. "Too many ghosts," she said. "I'm too sympathetic . . . I lose control . . . I'm no help to them because I can't shake my own grief and despair and sadness . . ." To the contrary, it is such circumstances that have the potential to make them ideal palliative caregivers, able to fully empathize and offer what they must know is needed. A few weeks after losing my twenty-five-year-old daughter in a sudden and violent tragedy, I returned and cared for a terminally ill child in the pediatric ICU. As I said to a stunned fellow nurse, "You just have to dive right back in, or the fear of reliving your heartache will prevent you from doing what you are called to do." Rather than burden patients' families with details of my own suffering, I simply let them know I was available to help them in their sorrow and that I had suffered a similar loss.

It is the rare patient who can accept his demise without a shred of emotion. I've often heard a chaplain ask patients if they know what's going to happen after they die. Only once did I hear the patient respond that yes, the sheets would be changed, the bed would be cleaned, and another patient would occupy his space.

Dr. Robert Bach, a palliative care physician called to his specialty only after losing his beloved wife of thirty-two years, is also a gifted poet. Having written extensively about loss, he reminds us that ignoring a person's loss in an effort "to spare him or her pain" is counterproductive. If one is to walk through the door to acceptance and healing, someone must first open it. Because memories are all that remain, these can be validated when shared. We are indebted to Dr.

Bach for sharing one of his poignant poems and communicating this concept in a very powerful way.

Stones in My Hand

As I stand watching the waves breaking on
the shore
I wonder why people don't talk about you
anymore

Perhaps they're afraid to stir up memories
of the past
But these are the very thoughts that I want to
always last

As I watch the ocean recede with the
outgoing tide
I fear that your spirit will be taken
from my side

As I sit on this rock and stare across
the bay
I try to listen and hear what you have
to say

There are no words but then a sudden warmth
I feel
And then I know for sure that your presence
is real

He has brought you with Him to be here
with me
And He has led me here to find you by
the sea

Each stone that I kneel down to pick up
and hold
Brings forth a memory that I want to
be told

My tears convey the words that my heart can
not say
And I know that I will meet you somewhere
every day

As I climb the steps, I feel the stones within
my hand
That once were meaningless just lying in
the sand

Subchapter 3: Memorable Patients

Helping another human being to die is as intimate an experience as helping another human to be born, and we are never ordinary souls after either.

Bill was a robust man of eighty-one years, with a balding head and long white sideburns. He had the biggest hands of any man I'd ever seen: hard-working hands, rugged, calloused, and huge by any standard. I looked over at the woman sitting in the chair by the window, and I asked her if this was her husband.

"We were married sixty-one years ago," she answered.

"What did he do for work?"

"He was a train conductor for the Bangor and Aroostook Railroad," she said proudly. "Bill drove the train from Searsport to Fort Kent."

The next day was a beautiful, sunny fall day. The leaves were at their peak brilliance of crimsons, golds, and oranges. This would be Bill's last day, one that would be detailed by Bill's wife in his obituary. Bill seemed to have accepted his fate.

"I wish I could take you with me," I overheard him say to his wife.

As a gentle breeze blew in through the open window, Bill's wife was drawn to the beauty of the river and trees below. She could make out an eagle roosting on a tree across the river and followed the outlines of the distant eddies as they emerged from the nearby dam. She could see the train tracks as they wound around the river and made their way past the hospital below, and she squeezed her husband's hand a little tighter. The train passed by the hospital every day at the same time, something we who worked there came to know by the chugging of the engine and the clanging of the freight cars. Now, a new sound pierced the air, shrill and beckoning. I looked out the window as the train's whistle sounded, something I'd not heard it do before. I looked at the clock: 2:20 pm. I didn't have to look down at the bed to know Bill had just drawn his last breath and answered the train's call.

"Always you have been told that work is a curse and labor a misfortune. But I say to you that when you work, you fulfill a part of Earth's furthest dream, assigned to you when that dream was born."
~Khalil Gibran, *The Prophet*

In the 1980s I researched and gave a lecture on near-death experiences. Karen, who was in the medical profession herself but did not know me at this time, claims it was the most intriguing lecture she'd ever attended. If attendance is any indicator, I guess it wasn't so bad, as there was standing room only in our largest auditorium by the end of the daylong program. In preparation, I had interviewed several people, including patients and hospital employees' wives who claimed to have experienced such phenomena. Wikipedia defines *near-death experiences* (*NDEs*) as "profound personal experiences associated with death or impending death which researchers claim share similar characteristics." They include out-of-body occurrences and are a little more intense than the near-death feelings we have each morning when our alarm clocks go off at 4:45. Little did I know that my research would prepare me for some otherwise inexplicable phenomena in my own patient encounters.

On a busy afternoon, I was called to help with the resuscitation of Peter, who had gone into a lethal cardiac arrhythmia before having his blood pressure fall dangerously low and passing out. I made my way through the throng of professionals who were gathering to assist. Looking at the monitor, I quickly assessed that the patient was in ventricular tachycardia, a deadly rhythm for which cardioversion by electrical shock is the best treatment. I placed the conductive pads on his chest, charged the defibrillator, yelled "Everyone clear!" and sent 120 joules of electricity coursing through his chest wall. It worked, and normal sinus rhythm was restored. The next step was to try and figure out what had caused the dangerous arrhythmia in the first place. All in all, we were in his room for thirty, perhaps forty, minutes.

Later that evening, before leaving work for the day, I visited Peter to see how he was doing. When I entered his room, he stared closely at me and declared, "Hey, you're the guy who threw me a lifeline from shore when I was drowning in the river."

Peter was unconscious during the period of time I'd been in the room earlier, and we hadn't met prior. Though approximately forty percent of such patients report having a near-death experience (if they are asked after resuscitation), they are usually hesitant to bring it up themselves, afraid of being labeled as *crazy*.

"I know you're telling me the truth," I said, "Because I can't swim."

Sometimes when I feel as if I am being asked to give more than I think I am able, I remember a beautiful young lady who taught me a lot about selflessness. She was a college student, who along with another young student had been trapped in a terrible fire. Her name was Anne.

Anne had the deepest, most beautiful blue eyes I'd ever seen. Except for a small area about the size of a quarter on her back, her eyes were the only areas of her body not ravaged in the fire. Third-degree burns on over eighty percent of one's body is generally associated with

172

high mortality. Her physician, who despite these odds wanted to feel useful, would come in and cut off the dead and blackened layers of skin.

One Friday evening just prior to her death, Anne asked me, "What are you going to do for fun this weekend?"

I choked back the lump in my throat. Looking into her eyes, I wondered if I could have asked such a selfless question had our roles been reversed.

"I used to complain that I didn't have any shoes, until I met
a man who didn't have any feet."
~Old Persian proverb

"And in the end, it's not the years in your life that count. It's
the life in your years."
~Abraham Lincoln, 16th president of the USA

St. Patrick's Day is all about the luck of the Irish. For me, it will also always be tied to the memory of a young lad by the name of Justin. He was all of five years old when he came to our pediatric unit with acute lymphoblastic leukemia (ALL), and he kept us all on our toes.

One day Nurse Zoey caught Justin picking his nose.

"Oh, that's nasty," Nurse Zoey began. "It can give you lots of germs."

Not to be caught in something disgusting by a beautiful chick, Justin quickly quipped, "I was just putting this one back in!"

When his father brought him a toy measuring tape, Justin was entertained for hours measuring everything he could and trying each time to find something a little bit bigger than a previous item he'd measured. When Nurse Zoey bent over, Justin quickly came up behind her, expanded the tape across the unsuspecting nurse's bottom, and declared, "Wow, twenty-five inches!"

To say Justin was loved would be an understatement. He won the hearts of all of us who cared for him. He made us laugh; he made us cry. We would never be quite the same again.

After a summer spent in and out of our unit on various treatments, physicians determined little Justin would need a bone marrow transplant. In order to be ready for the rigorous transplant protocol, in which immunity is pretty much wiped out, Justin returned to our unit in September in an effort to build up his strength.

"I met my kindergarten teacher last week," he told me one day.

"Oh yeah? Is she nice?"

"Yeah, she's pretty cool. She told me the Leprechauns sometimes come to her classroom when the kids aren't there, and the kids try to set traps to catch one of them. Last year, they almost got one, and they have his shoe to prove it!"

"That *is* pretty cool. How would *you* go about catching one?"

"I'd kick him in the nuts!"

Justin's father was a minister at the local Pentecostal church, and his mother was the Sunday school teacher there. She was sitting in the corner of the room reading a religious journal and peered at Justin over the top of her glasses, mortified by the words her son had used.

Picking up on her cue, I asked Justin if he could use gentler words.

He thought for a moment and answered, "I'd kick him in the balls!"

I winked at the mom, and she smiled.

"I told my teacher I could already count to one hundred and say my ABCs. I think she was pretty impressed with me."

"Great. When do you start?"

"You hafta get me strong, see? I really want to start with Drew. He's my best friend."

"We'll do our best. But you have to help too. Like eating all your peas and carrots. Okay?"

"Okay," and with a smile Justin hunkered down under his covers and drifted off to sleep.

The next morning, I came in just as the code cart was getting there. "There's a code in 877," someone quickly shouted to me.

Couldn't be, I thought to myself. *That's Justin's room. Please, God, no.*

A smiling, mischievous face looked up at me as I ran into the room. "Wow," he said. "This is more exciting than I thought it would be! When I asked the operator what a 'doctor, STAT' was, she just asked me what room I was in and I told her. Who are all these people, anyway?"

Faced with the alternative of a real *STAT* (the code word we used for a patient who was in respiratory and/or cardiac arrest, from the Latin word *statim*, which means "immediately"), I couldn't be angry with Justin. I know he probably fabricated some of the details of how this came to be, but it didn't matter. He was okay; I was okay; everything was okay.

As the weeks went on, it was obvious that getting Justin stronger would be an uphill battle. Everything he ate seemed to go right through him. By October, the decision to do the transplant was made despite his failing weight. We prepared him for his trip to Boston, which he would make the following day.

"Justin," I said. "There's something odd going on. I found this gold coin under your bed."

"Whoa! It must be a Leprechaun! This is our chance to catch one!"

"What a great idea! Yeah---let's do it!"

Justin and I spent much of the afternoon tying together an elaborate trap with materials supplied by our activities department.

175

When he was satisfied it would indeed do the job, we very carefully placed it under his bed and hooked it up to his call bell.

Justin was so excited at the prospect of catching one of the creatures that he forgot all about the trip he would make the next day. At 6:30 the following morning, he awoke to the sound of several of us nurses flooding into his room with the exciting news that Justin's trap had been successful. The call bell had gone off, and sure enough, we'd caught a Leprechaun!

"Can I see him?" the excited youngster asked.

"He made a deal with us. He promised that if we let him go immediately, he would bring some luck to you in Boston. And he left this other gold coin for you so you would know he meant it."

I never saw a happier face on any human than the one Justin wore on his way out of our unit for his trip to Boston. Several weeks later, we were told Justin had received his transplant. After a month in Boston, he came home, and pooling our resources, we sent him a large get-well card. We signed it, "Pat, the Leprechaun." We're told he treasured it and that he was a hero in the eyes of his classmates for the few short months he was able to attend kindergarten. Justin passed away on St. Patrick's Day due to relapse of the leukemia. As former caregivers, we were of course saddened; but we were also comforted by the fact that we'd helped to bring a little magic into a life that was otherwise out of our hands.

"Life's not always fair. Sometimes you can get a splinter even sliding down a rainbow."
~Terri Guillemets, author

Native American heritage in Maine is rich. The Penobscots (whose name means "the descending ledge place" and refers to the falls between Old Town and Bangor) are closely connected with the Abnaki, Passamaquoddy, Malecite, and Pennacook Tribes. They owe their language to the Algonquians and eventually lent their name to a bay, a river, and a county in the state of Maine, and they settled villages in what are now towns such as Passadumkeag, Kenduskeag, and Mattawamkeag. The Penobscot and Passamaquoddy Tribes constitute the only bodies of Native Americans of any size in New England.

By the time Maine became a state in 1820, the Penobscot Tribe had given up all of their ancestral lands and were left with their main village upriver from Bangor, called "Indian Old Town" by the settlers. Even this was eventually taken over by White settlers, who called it "Old Town" and pushed the Tribe farther across the river onto a seven-and-a-half-square-mile parcel of land, which became the Penobscot Indian Island Reservation. Today, we call it simply "Indian Island," and it is home to about six hundred people, twenty-three percent of whom live below the poverty level.

Not long after I first started working as a nurse, a Penobscot man arrived in our unit. Charlie had been found frozen and without a heartbeat. Doctors tried in vain to slowly rewarm his body. Ultimately, it remained in the position in which rigor mortis had claimed it---with his right arm extended at a ninety-degree angle out from his trunk. In the process of gathering his belongings, I started to pick up a feather lying next to him.

"White Man, don't touch Indian feather," a family member quickly said.

Looking up, I saw apprehension in the family member's eyes and dread in his trembling jaw. I had meant no disrespect, but the man's startled and horrified reaction caused me to pause and consider my misstep.

I recognized the look on his face as the same one I'd seen on the face of a young African American fellow VISTA volunteer, Lenny, I'd naively and unwisely taken to a Ku Klux Klan (KKK) rally in Lynchburg, Virginia years earlier. I'd been curious about what all the hubbub was about, thought I could stand up and tell them all that what they were doing was wrong, and told him where we were going. He was the same person whose trust I'd earned when we swapped roles one day, and he had come to believe me whenever I told him I would protect him. Still, when we drove into the park filled with white-hooded "priests" carrying torches, he looked at me incredulously, crouching and shivering in the well of the passenger side of my army truck with government plates.

Now, that look was written on this family member's face, and I knew the feather must have great significance. I said my condolences and withdrew to another room until the family member picked up the feather and left.

Later, I discovered that the feather is considered a sacred connection between the human and spirit worlds. The hollow shaft is thought to allow a person's prayers to rise up toward the heavens and to also conduct wisdom from the Great Spirit to his people. Birds are thought to be messengers between the two realms, which places further significance on the feather.

As I was returning to Charlie's room to make final preparations to transport him to the morgue, I passed through the waiting room to retrieve a message from the receptionist's desk. I noticed several of Charlie's family members sitting together and talking. They sat next to the desk, and it was hard not to overhear their words.

"You know that woman who was in here crying yesterday?"

"Yeah?"

"I found out she's the wife of the judge who gave Charlie a year with six months suspended for shoplifting. Seems he died."

Interesting, I thought, as I picked up my message and continued on my way. The job of transporting this poor fellow on a stretcher to the morgue fell upon me. Anticipating I would need help, I enlisted Nurse Miles. The morgue was only two buildings away, but navigating the basement connecting these buildings, with all its turns and narrow doorways, proved to be quite a feat. The arm needed constant attention to keep it from blocking an entrance or slapping someone coming in the opposite direction. Miles helped me turn Charlie on his side in these instances.

When we finally reached our destination, I noticed another patient, who had been transported to the morgue just the night before, still lying there. As I'd learned from Charlie's family member, the former patient had been a prominent judge who once gave this Native American patient an exorbitant prison sentence for a very petty crime. Now, ironically, the two were lying side by side as cellmates. The Great Spirit, it seems, had spoken.

"The glories of our blood and state
Are shadows, not substantial things;
There is no armor against Fate;
Death lays his icy hand on kings;
Scepter and Crown
Must tumble down,
And in the dust be equal made
With the poor crooked scythe and spade."
~ James Shirley, playwright, poet

In the early 1980s, not long after I started practicing nursing, the AIDS epidemic reared its ugly head. Its stigma was associated with a wave of repercussions, such as discrimination by insurance carriers and employers. In order to protect the rights of such patients, legal and medical practice reforms launched programs making it nearly impossible for anyone but the treating physician to know if a patient carried the virus predisposing them to the deadly disease. (If the human immunodeficiency virus is present, the patient is said to be "HIV positive.") Although caregivers practiced *universal precautions*, meaning that everyone was treated as potentially contagious, there were circumstances when a definitive diagnosis would have been helpful. In those days, lab reports were not computerized but were available on paper. I voiced my concern to one of the physicians, Dr. W, who frequented the ICU in those days.

"There's an easy way to know," he said.

"Really? How?" I asked eagerly.

"If I put the patient's lab report in the recycling bin, the result is 'negative.' If I put it in my pocket, the patient is 'HIV positive.'"

A few weeks later, I saw Dr. W pocket a lab report. Sidney had come in with Kaposi's sarcoma, a common finding in patients with final stage AIDS, and I was not surprised about the diagnosis. I knew it would be only a matter of days before the young man would be put on mechanical support, and I watched for an opportune time to help him sort out his final wishes.

"Am I going to die?" he asked me the next day.

"It doesn't look good, Sidney." Unless a caregiver is straightforward with such a patient, the patient may never again have the opportunity to express whatever he needs to say. He took a few moments to compose himself, and then continued with things he'd obviously been considering.

"If you could notify my sister, it would be a huge load off my mind," he began. "She's the only family I've got left, and I haven't been very good about keepin' in touch with her the last few years. Sure would like to say goodbye to her at least."

He gave me her telephone number and thanked me for being honest. After giving Sidney his afternoon meds, I made the difficult call. His sister didn't waste any time in coming, and they spent the rest of that day and all of the next reminiscing about their years growing up and catching up on the few years they'd been apart. Then he lay back, closed his eyes, and went to sleep.

Respiratory distress was followed by respiratory failure over the next few hours, and Sidney's doctor made the decision to intubate him. The next day Sidney suffered an intracerebral bleed. He was pronounced brain dead thirty-six hours later, his sister by his side. As I removed the wires and tubes connecting him to the breathing machine, I watched in horror as Sidney raised his right arm and put his hand to his mouth. I quickly excused myself to Sidney's sister and found the doctor still at the ICU nursing station.

"I think we made a mistake," I said to the physician. "He couldn't have been dead." I recounted what happened, but the physician just stared at me without saying a word. While I was thinking we should resuscitate the poor man, the doctor was looking at me as if I needed to double up on my psych meds (which I hadn't considered taking before this happened). I eventually went back and finished cleaning up my patient, feeling that I must quit my addiction to coffee.

Not long after my apparent hallucination, however, I heard about a man who, just prior to being embalmed, sat bolt upright on the undertaker's table. Armed with this new evidence, I sat down at my computer and researched the possibility of such occurrences. The *Lazarus sign*, named, of course, after the most famous person to have been raised from the dead by Jesus, is a real phenomenon. Just as chickens can run around with their heads cut off, severe lack of oxygen and blood in tissues can set off a firing of spinal motor neurons that can result in such involuntary movements in humans. I breathed a satisfied sigh of relief, picked up my cup, and headed for the coffee pot.

In mid-October of 1986, my neighbor Glen was admitted to ICU. I was saddened to learn Glen was in the late stages of pancreatic cancer. We always looked forward to going to Glen's house during Halloween, and it wasn't because he and his wife gave out generous handfuls of candy. In fact, at Glen's house, you helped yourself.

Glen lived in a yellow raised ranch situated down a long driveway. On the left side lay a detached garage, and on the right side was a walkway to the front porch and the front door. Glen always left the light on over the front porch, so that the children could navigate their way up the two steps and find the large dish of Baby Ruths, Nestle's Crunch Bars, and Three Musketeers he would set out.

The first year I brought Jodie and Jane trick-or-treating in his neighborhood, I told them I would watch from the road while they went to Glen's house. We'd walked a fair distance by then, and my feet needed a break. Glen and his wife had done a great job decorating for the occasion. A haystack hugged the mailbox, pumpkins carved into lighted jack-o'-lanterns lined the walkway, and a pumpkin-headed scarecrow sat limply on the porch, its straw hands encircling the great dish of candy. I pulled the collar of my jacket closer to my head, feeling the wind pick up a bit and the temperature drop with the sun's setting. A rustling in the trees surrounding the house broke the silence, and my girls laughed at their being startled by a squirrel. They merrily made their way up the steps and onto the porch, where they read a simple note above the candy dish: "Take some if you dare."

"No problem," Jane, my younger and more adventurous girl said. She began to fill her bag with her favorite candy bars. Then something odd happened. The scarecrow started to move. It grabbed at the children's hands, stood up, and began to chase the girls in floppy, ineffective movements. The girls, of course, were stunned. They screamed and ran off the porch and down the driveway into my waiting arms.

"We better get out of here," I said, playing along with Glen's prank.

The following year, my older girl Jodie wanted nothing to do with Glen's house. She'd had enough of being frightened. But Jane loved thrills and adventure and talked her older sister into accompanying her down the driveway.

"Besides," she observed. "There's no scarecrow this year. Look."

Sure enough, the scarecrow that had guarded the candy the year before was gone. The great bowl of chocolate delights was sitting on a table under the porch light. The other decorations from the year prior seemed harmless.

I watched from the road again as my girls stepped onto the porch more vigilantly this time. They looked around and then began to fill their bags. Suddenly, they heard a noise. It seemed to be coming from under their feet. Sure enough, the pumpkin-headed scarecrow appeared from beneath the porch and again began to pursue them in his clumsy fashion. It was a narrow escape.

Curiosity is a powerful thing. Jane dragged Jodie back to Glen's house for a third year. Though Jane and I were enjoying this immensely, Jodie could have done without the excitement and talked me into walking halfway down the driveway to wait for them. They peered under the porch with their flashlights before climbing the steps.

"Coast is clear!" shouted Jane, and they eagerly scurried up the steps and began to fill their bags, their backs to the walkway and garage, looking at each other with a sense of relief that they seemed to be in the clear. But this was not to be. With a great crash, the overhead garage door opened, and in the lighted garage entrance stood the figure of a great Frankensteinish monster. It held out its arms toward the girls and slowly dragged great, clanging chains behind it. Though it was great entertainment for me, I tried to hide my amusement and keep things serious as the girls came shrieking back.

"I sure enjoyed Halloween," Glen said, as we sat reminiscing. "I'm going to miss dressing up and playing with the kids."

"Those were good times," I agreed, taking a pink capsule from my scrub coat pocket and handing it to Glen with a glass of water. "This is just Dalmane, something to help you sleep. Oops, on second thought, give that back to me. I gave you one of my Good 'N Plenty licorice bites by mistake. This is the *right* one."

In fact, we were the ones left to miss Glen. His wife told me they'd always wanted children of their own but were never blessed with any. After Glen died, the neighborhood was never quite the same at Halloween. The Mrs. still puts out a pumpkin-headed scarecrow, but it just doesn't seem to have the same spunk as in years past.

Skydiving has become a popular sport for thrill-seekers. The ecstasy one gets from hurtling one's body from thirteen thousand feet above Earth at 115 miles per hour prior to reaching chute pull altitude is often touted as the ultimate high. For one thirty-two-year-old man, the sport would prove life-changing. He was brought to the ER in 2002 upon suffering injuries after his damaged canopy landed him in a tree. Though the branches cushioned his fall and probably saved his life, a large stick pierced the tiny gap separating the face shield from the rest of the helmet and impaled him through the left eardrum. The stick penetrated roughly eight inches of the man's brain.

"I'd like to request a DNR order for Mr. Harvey." I looked up and saw that a woman had made her way to the nursing station and was standing over me.

"Mr. Harvey?" I asked, somewhat taken aback by her boldness and unable to place the name.

"You haven't got him yet. He's on his way in from the emergency room."

A few areas of nursing may come naturally to some, but to others—like me—these areas required funneling through the school of hard knocks to get them to solidify. One such area was the timing of the discussion with families (or, rarely in our unit, patients) about Do Not Resuscitate (DNR) orders. Medical personnel are aware that people can and do sometimes die in a hospital, and resuscitation is attempted on all patients *unless* a DNR is requested. Early in my career, a young doctor gave me a tongue-lashing about talking to a patient about his DNR status; this role, he asserted, was reserved for the physician. An older physician, upon overhearing this, suggested to his younger colleague that such a discussion was just an invitation for a dialogue. Out of the 1440 minutes of each day a patient is in the unit, a doctor may spend ten minutes with the patient. It would seem only natural for a family to open such a door with the nurses, who see the patient the other 1430 minutes and know more intimately the details of the patient's suffering. Today, it is common practice for the nurse to take the lead in having such a dialogue.

I also reasoned that the nurse spends a miniscule amount of time with the patient compared with the time their loved ones have spent with them outside the hospital, and that this criterion should make them eligible to be in the room during resuscitation efforts. I welcomed them into the space, maintaining they were the most important persons in the room. Many other nurses were less enthusiastic about allowing this, and I soon learned to yield to the wishes of the patient's primary nurse, who knows the family best and who can judge the appropriateness of allowing this.

In the olden days, Grandma took one last gasp, and that was the end of it. But now, with all the new technology available, a patient dies bit by bit. If the lungs fail, she is put on a machine that breathes for her. If she suffers a heart attack while on the ventilator, she can be put on a cardiac assist device. If the kidneys begin to fail, she is connected to a dialysis machine to cleanse her blood. And if the liver fails, a tube can be inserted into the liver vein to decrease the pressure. At each step, machines *aid* in helping the patient survive to endure the next. And this is the real crux of the dilemma: at what point do the efforts of prolonging the patient's life become tools in prolonging her death? Indeed, the fear of *death* is being replaced by the fear of *dying these high-tech deaths.*

Philosophically, it's easier to initiate a new treatment than it is to discontinue one of these treatments once it's in place. In the earlier days, one even needed a court order to remove someone from a ventilator. The decision to institute a DNR order should come only after careful consideration, ideally by the patient, of all aspects of the patient's prognosis and expected quality of life following a successful resuscitation. If a patient has not made such a determination regarding life-saving heroics, the family is usually in the next best position to make such a decision. Knowing when to have a frank discussion with the family is crucial.

In the case of the injured skydiver, a family member making such a request for a DNR so soon was highly unusual. Sensing something was not quite right, I took the woman's name and told her I would get back to her. She turned out to be the wife of the skydiver, and he turned out to be an alcoholic who had physically and emotionally abused her for years. She also reported he'd been hard of hearing, something that wasn't likely to get any better now.

I noted with approval that a most celebrated neurosurgeon and friend, Dr. King, was assigned to this case, and I chuckled, recalling an adventure we had shared the week before. Dr. King, who had set out to buy a barbecue grill for a family gathering, finally located a suitable one at the new big-box store with the orange and black sign near the mall. But he was daunted by the fact the grill needed to be assembled.

"Is there someone in Home Depot who could assemble this for me?" he asked the young man assisting him.

"No, but don't worry," he was told. "You won't have any trouble. It doesn't take a brain surgeon to put this together."

Being that the working parts of a grill and those of a brain have little in common, poor Dr. King struggled for several hours with the task until finally giving in and calling me over to assist. He was never too proud to admit when he needed help.

Within an hour of the skydiver's admission, Dr. King arrived to have a look with his *prospectoscope* (a term one of his colleagues, Dr. Dinerman, had coined a few years earlier). He'd seen his share of unusual trauma cases and knew there was no need to rush into a decision about either the prognosis or the DNR.

"I'd like to consult with another neurosurgeon about this. Let's keep him on the antibiotics until then."

Dr. King had consulted with the second neurosurgeon on another case in the late 1970s. Their patient was diagnosed with a rare pituitary tumor, and surgery to remove it was something with which neither of them had any prior experience. It required an incision be made just inside the area where the upper lip connects with the gum line. Access to the pituitary gland, which sits between one's eyes, is then made using a transsphenoidal approach by tunneling up through the base of the nose. It was a scary proposition, and neither surgeon felt very comfortable with it. As luck would have it, there was a deceased patient in the morgue who had no family and no identity. "In the name of medicine," the two surgeons performed the surgical procedure on the deceased woman without a hitch and found it only fitting to then pay for her pauper's grave. They later successfully applied what they'd learned to Dr. King's tumor patient.

Dr. King now found himself in another delicate case. The stick had penetrated a region of the brain considered *non-eloquent*, which means it was not needed to sustain speech, motor functions, and senses. There would, however, be considerable debris, and the risk of infection could not be overstated. By the next day, the two physicians agreed to do the surgery together and scheduled it for the following morning.

As we were preparing our sedated patient for surgery, I noticed on the man's thigh a large tattoo of a Nazi Swastika. I recalled the wife's request and was struck by the cycle of violence that had apparently enveloped this man's life.

"Oh, that's really weird," I commented.

Nurse Brooke, his primary nurse, read the disgust in my face and said, "His parents probably didn't love him enough. He probably felt companionship from his Nazi fanatic friends and from the alcohol, companionship he felt he couldn't get anywhere else."

Brooke was a young rookie, but her words were those of someone who was all too familiar with such sadness.

"You're right, Brooke," I said. "Who am I to judge?"

Though the surgery was long and tedious, the results were spectacular, and the request for a DNR order was denied. Who could

188

have predicted someone with a stick through his head could have lived and done well? Modern medicine has come close to turning out miraculous transformations; social reform has a bit of catching up to do.

Subchapter 4: Putting It All Together: A Memorable and Enduring Impact

"Lying awake, calculating the future, trying to unweave, unwind, unravel and piece together the past and the future, between midnight and dawn, when the past is all deception, the future futureless. . ."
~T. S. Eliot

In the course of every nurse's career, there is bound to be one or two patients who stand out. Of the thousands of patients I encountered, Daryl was one of those patients. He embodied every emotion of any patient with whom I ever worked, presented more challenges than any of the others, and forced me to hone my skills and grow my talents more than anyone else. Like the games of chess we sometimes shared with each other to pass the time during his eight-month stay from December of 1984 to August of 1985, each of his *moves* required a special *move* from me. It proved to be a time that would test our wills and our faiths, a time that would forever change our lives, and a time that would join us in a lasting bond of friendship. We are indebted to him for providing his thoughts (in bold font) and encourage readers who would like to read more about Daryl's ordeal to obtain his excellent booklet, *Passing Showers*[13], excerpts of which appear here in italicized font.

He came to us in a state of severe muscle weakness, his large, six-foot-and-two-inch frame useless against the monster that was enveloping it. He had Guillain-Barré Syndrome (GBS), and without a doubt the worst case I would ever see. GBS is a disorder in which the body's immune system attacks parts of the nervous system. Such an attack leads to nerve inflammation, which in turn causes tingling, muscle weakness, and paralysis. The specific trigger is unknown, but GBS usually follows a minor infection. Though it most often affects the nerve's covering, which results in signals that move more slowly, GBS can also damage other parts of the nerve, which can cause the nerve to stop working altogether. The condition progresses very rapidly, and it may take only a few hours to reach the most severe symptoms.

In Daryl's case, he had awoken one morning after a bout with the flu and was immediately aware of severe weakness in his legs, eventually losing the ability to stand unassisted. By the time he arrived in our unit, the paralysis had started to ascend to his arms. We worked quickly to prepare for artificial ventilation support, which would likely be needed in the event his breathing muscles were affected.

For the average man, this would indeed present a great challenge. But Daryl was no ordinary man; he was a man of God, a minister of faith. When I read his chart on my way into his room on our first day together, I made it a point to read all the demographics:

Occupation: minister
Marital Status: married
Children: three
Age: 34.

I looked at the tall, handsome man who was by this time staring back at me, and I introduced myself, resisting in the final instant the urge to offer my handshake. Sitting in the corner of the room was Daryl's wife of eleven years, Mary, a lovely woman with a quick and gentle smile. On her lap sat the youngest of their three boys. Though I did not want to frighten them any more than they already were, I also knew if the paralysis continued to his breathing muscles and Daryl lost his ability to speak for any period of time, we would need to have an alternate means of communication in place.

"Hello," I began. I knew this would be a long haul, and I sat down.

Mary presented a very calm, dedicated and helpful demeanor. She helped answer my questions without hesitation, knowing her responses would be useful in helping her husband through this terrible ordeal.

"Do *you* have any questions about this condition?" I finally asked, afraid of the tough questions that might result but willing to research any answers I didn't readily have. The diagnosis of GBS would not be final until later in the day, when the results of the spinal tap and electromyogram would be ready. I tried to provide information that was applicable to most neuropathies.

Mary glanced at Daryl and then back at me, and I anticipated she was asking this one for him. "Will he get better?"

I knew about ninety percent of patients with GBS survive and recover completely, though it might take years. I also knew a good outcome was predicted if the symptoms abated within three weeks. "It's really too soon to know," I answered, and I described the possible scenarios and prepared her for the possible complications. Besides the respiratory failure which he now faced, Daryl was at risk for deep vein thrombosis and skin ulcers due to his inactivity, pneumonia and other infections, an unstable blood pressure, and permanent paralysis.

That afternoon, I received a phone call from Daryl's father, who was calling from Pennsylvania and wanted to come to visit his son. He needed to tend to some business before leaving and wanted some idea about how long Daryl would be in the hospital. He also needed to know how much he and his wife should pack. Things did not look good. What could I say?

"I would plan for Daryl to be in the hospital for eight to ten months," I said. I felt that should cover the worst-case scenario. There was silence on the other end. Daryl's father was in shock. "Please know we will do everything possible to get your son better." I later learned Daryl's father was shocked that a nurse, rather than a doctor, was able to tell him such information. In the end, my prediction was right on the mark.

"Hi there." I winked at the young boy who sat at Daryl's bedside. "Could you help your father out by getting me a mouth swab from the drawer next to you?" Involving the family in the patient's care is quite therapeutic, and the youngster eagerly jumped up and proudly handed me the swab. He smiled at his dad, who winked quickly to ward off a tear.

"Daryl, we need to prepare for the worst in case it happens. If the paralysis ascends high enough to render you without the ability to speak, we're going to need a system whereby you can still communicate. If you are connected to a ventilator, you will not be able to use your voice. Think about what might work well for you, and I'll be back in a few moments to work out the details with you."

By the time I got back to Daryl a few minutes later, he and Mary had worked out a clever, albeit tedious, scheme of spelling and blinking through the alphabet one letter at a time. We worked on shortening the procedure by blinking once for "yes" and twice for "no" to questions such as narrowing down the location of the letter to the beginning or ending half of the alphabet or to whether the letter he was going for was a consonant or a vowel. *Wheel of Fortune*, eat your heart out!

Not long afterward, a measurement of his vital capacity signaled it was time to provide him with breathing support. Vital capacity measurements are an indication of the volume of breath one can take in and breathe out; a vital capacity of 800 cc per breath signals that action is needed. Within twenty-four hours after the first symptoms had appeared, Daryl found himself on a ventilator. Within a week, he found himself sealed within a prison of nearly complete paralysis. His eyes and his eyelids were the only muscles spared. As Daryl would later write, *In many ways, it was if I had been buried alive right there amidst the tubes and machines and monitors crammed over and around my hospital bed.* I wrote the blinking instructions on a piece of paper and hung them on the wall as a reminder to staff and to Daryl: one blink for "yes;" two blinks for "no."

So, for many long weeks and months, I was almost completely paralyzed — fully alert, but unable to move my fingers, toes, legs, arms, and neck muscles. Even my facial muscles were paralyzed, so I could not smile or frown . . . The ventilation tube connected with my windpipe below my larynx, so it was impossible for me to speak or even whisper. Neither could I swallow, stretch, shift my weight, or call for help.

Weeks later, when I was finally once again able to begin turning my head from side to side, someone taped a call bell to my pillow so that I could roll my head onto it. The idea was meritorious, but the tape would often loosen or the button would shift on the pillow, rendering me once again totally helpless to even call for a nurse.

Mary visited and prayed every day, bringing the three boys when she could. Still, Daryl's progress was disappointing. Many of the therapeutic interventions in vogue today, such as plasmapheresis, which can help limit the severity of the disease, were just coming into use in 1984. Since then, we have learned how critical the timing of such techniques is. By the end of the first three weeks, Daryl could twitch his nose.

"Good morning, Daryl," I said one morning not long after the three-week mark had been reached. "Do you want to go for a ride?" It was just after Christmas, and I thought seeing all the window paintings done by staff would help lift his spirits.

Two blinks told me I had my work cut out for me. As Daryl stared at me, I thought I could hear his voiceless thoughts screaming, "Leave me alone! I don't want your help or your pity---let me die---please let me die!"

I looked at Mary, and she smiled and shrugged her shoulders. She lowered the copy of *Why Us: When Bad Things Happen to God's People*, which she'd been reading to her husband. Having cared for many other quadriplegics before Daryl, I was all too familiar with such a scene. Self-pity is rampant in such cases, and it is always a challenge to help the patient find a purpose in life. Daryl's father told me that prior to his illness, Daryl had been a very organized man, who enjoyed control over every aspect of his life. Suddenly, he had become totally dependent upon all those around him. I tucked that important tidbit of background information away for the time being, but it would become the basis for many of my interventions over the coming months.

As if to remind staff of his circumstances, Daryl learned to "cluck" repeatedly with his tongue, a technique he blamed on the ingenuity of a respiratory therapist (RT). He preferred this to the call-bell setup I had improvised for him because it was easier and, I think, because it forced everyone else to notice and to share in the pervasiveness of his suffering. He clucked for any little thing every five minutes, perhaps a hundred times a shift. Daryl needed his pillow readjusted, he needed to be turned onto his side, or onto his back, or onto his side again. He needed his pain meds. We knew he was just scared and lonely. Just as fathers tend to play down and ignore whining and mothers tend to give in and pamper, we male nurses were inclined to answer only the call-bell signals, which we interpreted as more urgent, while the female nurses went running to Daryl's every cluck. When we recently asked Daryl if he remembered this communication technique, he had a more light-hearted take on events.

Now, as to whether I was a clucker. Neither Mary nor I were certain about what a clucker is, but I don't think I particularly like the sound of it.

Mary thought maybe it's someone on a vent who makes loud mouth sounds to get attention. If so, I'm afraid I'm guilty. But Debbie the RT gets part of the blame for that. She taught me how to snap my tongue off the roof of my mouth in a way that made such a loud sound people could hear it in the lobby. I even had reports people could hear it out on State Street on a quiet night.

Anyway, it worked. Nurses would come running from all over the hospital. At first, I thought they were genuinely concerned about whether I was okay. But then I noticed Ray and Leon and other male nurses never responded. It was just the girls, and especially the most attractive female nurses who came and ACTED concerned. But it soon became apparent they actually just enjoyed my company — you know, being in my room, in my presence — and were just using the clucking thing as an excuse to come in and spend time with me. At that point Mary put an end to the whole thing and forbid me to do any more clucking and clacking.

These scenes were played out repeatedly over the first three months. In an attempt to get him out of his bed and keep him in our sights, we asked Daryl if he wanted to sit out at the nursing station and watch us work. What we really wanted him to do was to socialize, to overcome a condition that patients on bed rest in ICU for a long time often succumb to: "ICU-itis," as we often referred to it. Daryl always resisted. For a long time, we would ask and be put off. After a while, we just started getting him up without asking *if* he wanted to, but instead asking *which side of*

195

the bed he wanted us to get him out of. He would sit for hours and watch the activity, accompanied by his oxygen tank and a ventilator or ambu bag (hand bagger). At first, once set up there, he constantly clucked to get a nurse to take him back to his room. Later, he seemed to look forward to it.

The care I received was great, but being a patient in an ICU for an extended period of time can cause problems of its own.

First, the limited number of windows in the ICU made it difficult to know what time of the day it was. Days and nights soon began to merge and time became one long, seemingly endless, blur of monotonous misery.

The ICU also made it impossible to see visitors — except for my immediate family. My interaction with the outside world and any sense of normal life routine was filtered through the ICU staff and a few of my closest family members.

I've often wondered if visiting-hour rules, including the screening of potential visitors, are formulated with the nurse or with the patient in mind, and it's always been my contention that the uniqueness of family situations begs that the patient, rather than the hospital, should determine who might visit.

Perhaps the greatest challenge I faced was the loss of my ability to independently decide, influence, or control even many of the smallest of circumstances. I was almost completely dependent on others for everything.

For instance, when I was cold, I had to ask for a cover. When I was sore, I had to ask to be turned. When I needed to move my bowels, I had to ask for a bedpan. When I wanted to escape and be left alone, there was nowhere to run or hide. When I needed company or distraction, there were almost no options.

No options, that is, until one day one of my nurses proposed a way to address the problem.

Ray Buyno, R.N., was one of a number of ICU charge nurses who were assigned to my case. Nurse-patient dynamics are probably no different than many other human relationships. Sometimes a student will connect well with a teacher, and sometimes not. Sometimes a salesman will rub a buyer the wrong way and sometimes not. The same is true for lawyers and their clients, clerks and their customers, and so on.

Ray Buyno and I seemed to hit it off well from the beginning. Perhaps it was his sense of humor, his practical no-nonsense way of tackling problems, or his willingness to share principles from his own personal experiences. I suspect the one thing that made more of a difference than anything else was Ray's ability to put himself in his patients' situation, sense what we were experiencing, and then develop some sort of creative solution unique to the case.

Over four months of ICU isolation, staring at one spot on the ceiling, a lack of sunshine and fresh air, an almost total loss of independence, fear about the future, and significant sleep deprivation had all taken their toll. I was increasingly edgy, restless, depressed, irritable, and introspective.

That was the situation when one day Ray Buyno came into my room and announced, "I've got a little surprise for you today; something different."

In a few minutes, with help from a number of other nurses, he had gotten me out of bed and into a big recliner-on-wheels he'd apparently confiscated from some other part of the hospital. He then pushed me out beside the nursing station where he went back to work on his charts.

So, there I was, suddenly sitting just a few feet away from the nerve center of a busy ICU. I was still connected to the big Bear respirator but now, for the first time in months, I had a whole range of new sights and sounds and smells and sensory data coming my way.

In some ways it was just a small move, but it had an immense and immediate effect on my spirits. Now I was distracted from many of my own problems. Now I was sitting up, viewing the world from a *vertical* orientation. Now I was feeling more like a normal human being. Some of the doctors and others passing through the Unit would glance at me and say hello. It was as if I was once again almost a regular person.

I'm sure I was not the first or the last patient who Ray Buyno and his fellow nurses parked in a chair beside the nursing station. But at the time, I felt I was particularly privileged. It was almost as though someone had appointed me chief of the ICU for a few hours — supervising and monitoring a staff that was busy monitoring others.

Of course, that's not the way it actually was, but it's the way I *felt* it was for a little while. And I think it was finally being able to *feel* more normal that provided me with the boost necessary to continue on down the road to healing and actual normalcy.

By the end of March, anticipating Daryl would need to redirect his attention even further from the prison in which his physical impairment had landed him, I brought in a magnetic chess board from home and began "enjoying" chess strategies with him. I would make a move and then go about my business of caring for the other patients. Upon my return twenty minutes later, I would ask Daryl if he wanted this man to move or this one or this. And the same procedure was used to pinpoint the spot to which he wanted the piece to move. I must confess, being the poor player and even poorer sport that I was, I sometimes avoided offering a spot if I saw the move would get me trapped. This, of course, took a long time and required patience.

One of the most difficult aspects of my ordeal with Guillain-Barré syndrome (GBS) was the challenge of not giving in to a vicious cycle of introspection, fear, and frustration.

The extensive paralysis that marked my stay in the intensive care unit significantly narrowed my world. I was unable to walk or talk or open a book or use a computer. I was unable to hold a conversation or ventilate my frustration verbally. I couldn't cough up mucous, blow my nose, or wipe my eyes. Time inched by like a lazy slug all day long and especially at night.

Because I was unable to distract myself with external stimuli, my focus often turned inward. And the more I would think about my own physical discomfort, the more anxious and miserable I would become.

One night, while he was on duty as my nurse, Ray Buyno came into my room and said, "Hey, man, what's your favorite game? Do you like to play cards?" "No." "Do you like to play Scrabble?" "No." "How about Clue?" "No way."

Finally, when he mentioned chess, I begrudgingly consented.

"So, you're pretty good at chess, huh? You think you can beat me at chess? Okay, well, we'll see how that goes." And in a few minutes, he was back with a chess board.

Ray had many other responsibilities that night, with me and with other patients, so, as I recall, it took over an hour for him to even get the chess board set up and make the first move. He then asked me how I wanted to move my pieces, made the move for me, and left the room. Twenty-five more minutes went by before he returned.

Daryl likes to remind me that whenever he made a move that proved difficult for me, I seemed suddenly to have an urgent need to attend to another patient.

Over the next few hours, he only ever managed about three more moves for each of us. It was the slowest, most unsatisfactory, game of chess I had ever played. In fact, I don't think we ever did complete the game. And, although we played chess on several other occasions, I don't recall that we *ever* completed a game.

Perhaps that wasn't the point. What seemed to matter more was that I was distracted — at least to some extent — from my own physical problems. I was playing chess with Ray Buyno, the ICU charge nurse for whom I had developed a great deal of respect. There was a victory all of its own in that — a strategy I'm sure Ray must have had in mind long before the game ever started.

About this same time, I also asked another quadriplegic to come and talk to Daryl about life with paralysis. I like to think that seeing someone else in the same condition who was able to live a fruitful life might have given him hope. Though the cutoff beyond which patients are not expected to improve is usually given as one year, I thought it would be wise to prepare for the worst.

When April came, I felt we needed to up the challenge a bit, as I knew Daryl could not continue in his complacency. His father's words about previously having control in his life continued to direct my actions. In hindsight, I was being cocky and would probably not have proceeded this way now. The three boys smiled up at me one day in anticipation, as they had become accustomed to seeing me do some trick or tell some entertaining story. I asked Nurse Rachel to come in and gave her three cafeteria coupons. "Please take the boys for a little snack. You don't mind, do you, Mary?" She shook her head and smiled.

"Daryl," I began, not knowing exactly how I might proceed but trusting God would give me the words. Just then, the reporter for the local news on the television Daryl had been watching interrupted me with the slogan, "Big A---All the Way." *Thank you, God,* I whispered.

During my five-month stay in the intensive care unit (ICU) at Eastern Maine Medical Center (EMMC) with Guillain-Barré syndrome (GBS) in 1984-1985, a political drama was playing itself out in the Northwoods of Maine.

A huge hydroelectric development plan had been proposed by developers. If approved, the plan would have authorized the construction of two dams on the St. John River. One of the results of these dams being constructed would have been the flooding of the lower Allagash, a famed waterway championed then and now by conservationists and recreational advocates.

So, the battle was joined. Tensions were running high and the newspapers were filled with heated debate over how and when this matter would be settled.

One slogan that became particularly popular in the midst of the debate was: "Big A — All the Way!" Of course, "A" stood for Allagash and the slogan was everywhere — on bumper stickers, in TV ads, and even on roadside signs.

Meanwhile, I was lying in a hospital bed, completely paralyzed, trying to deal with the greatest trauma of my 34 years of life. Everything in my world had suddenly changed. It seemed all of the foundations had been ripped out from under me. And I was having a difficult time adjusting to all the changes — or even knowing if I *wanted* to adjust.

At first, I had tried to wait out the ordeal, hoping relief would come. But as the weeks turned to months, not much improvement was evident. So, I began to withdraw. Then I began to become fearful, irritable, and angry.

Of course, my bad-tempered response did not change the circumstances either, and even made matters worse. The whole ordeal began to take its toll on my family and on the medical staff. On one occasion my belligerent, insulting conduct and sentiments even resulted in a nurse leaving the ICU in tears. Something had to change.

Ray Buyno, R.N., was primarily responsible for my care plan at the time. One evening when he was in my room, the local newscast began covering the story of the Allagash project. Someone was citing the phrase "Big A — All the Way!" and at that moment Ray suddenly shut off the television and said, "I think it's time to tell you the truth. This whole Big A deal is just a giant publicity stunt cooked up for your sake. Did you know that? Big A doesn't really stand for Allagash; it stands for Acceptance, and this has all been promoted in an attempt to persuade you to accept the difficult circumstances now in your life."

With that Ray proceeded to lecture me for approximately ten minutes on all of the reasons why I should accept what had happened to me instead of fighting it. If I continued to refuse to accept what no one could change, he said, I was only going to end up digging myself into an even deeper hole.

Of course, I knew he was just fooling about the Big A story being a publicity stunt. But I also knew he was NOT fooling about the need for me to change my attitude.

Many tough days, weeks, and months followed. But I still clearly recall that night's exchange in Room 145. I have thought about it many times. And I believe in those critical moments, using a little humor as fertilizer, Ray sowed seeds that eventually grew into principles that helped me to deal with my disability more realistically.

A good nurse has to be an excellent medical caregiver. A *great* nurse has to be part counselor, part psychiatrist, part pastor, and part humorist — *and* an excellent medical caregiver. That evening Ray Buyno was a truly great nurse.

Acceptance was a very hard pill to swallow for someone who'd been in such control of his life. I decided to improvise a system to give Daryl a little more control over his circumstances.

"I'm going to let you feed yourself tonight," I said one evening. "I'm pretty busy."

He looked incredulously at me, for he still had no movement below the nipple line and no fine motor movements whatsoever. With brows knit together in scrutiny, he watched as I assembled a fifteen-foot piece of tubing and supported it in the grasp of a mechanical arm I had scrounged from another piece of equipment and placed by his head. It required him to move his head forward and to suck on it like a straw. The other end of the tubing was submerged in a fairly large container of warm bouillon. It worked and gave Daryl another baby step of independence.

By summertime, Daryl was still trying to exert control over the nurses. Instead of a bath, he insisted on a shower one day from Nurse Pam and Nurse Courtney on one of my days off. Pam finally gave in, donned a plastic garbage bag over her uniform, and helped Daryl into the shower. Score another victory, albeit a crazy one, for Daryl.

Not long after Daryl got off the ventilator and was transferred to one of the other floors, Dr. T recommended Daryl go see a psychiatrist. When he declined, a psychiatrist came in to see Daryl. Afterwards, Daryl confided in me that the psychiatrist had recommended to Mary that she leave Daryl, that she divorce him because he was "so depressed, angry, rough, and mean . . . and a quadriplegic." Mary, of course, would be the last woman on Earth to leave her husband, even in such a state. She is a very strong and devoted woman, who has been his earthly sustaining support during the thirty-nine years since his ordeal, and she understood that he was still the same kind, gentle, compassionate, and understanding man she had married.

When someone for whom faith is an important part of life encounters major physical adversity, the spiritual implications are also significant.

For years I had been a minister, accustomed to visiting people in the hospital. I had been a preacher who routinely encouraged others to trust God in difficult times. Now, suddenly, *I* was the patient, and *I* was in need of encouragement.

> But what if I should discover
> that the least among them all,
> the poorest of all the beggars,
> the most impudent of all the offenders,
> the very enemy himself—
> that these are within me,
> and that I myself stand in need
> of the alms of my own kindness—
> that I myself am the enemy
> who must be loved—what then?
> ~ C. G. Jung[14], psychiatrist

The emotional, psychological, and spiritual turmoil I encountered during my eight months at Eastern Maine Medical Center in 1984-1985 was in many ways more difficult than the physical part of that ordeal.

The fact that the vast majority of the hospital staff was sensitive to that fact helped immensely. With only a few (awful) exceptions, the doctors, nurses, Respiratory Therapists, Physical Therapists, and even housekeepers, allowed me to be human, and never implied that, because I was a minister by profession, I should somehow be above the doubts and questions and frustrations of others.

I will always be grateful for those who accepted me in spite of my various failures at coping well.

I will also always be grateful for the medical staff who prayed with me and listened to my bitter ramblings without condemning me.

And I will also always be very grateful for the many provisions that were in place to help me deal with the spiritual part of my struggle, e.g., the ready availability of hospital chaplains; permission for my church elders to enter the ICU one day and pray over me; the chapel services to where I was taken in a wheelchair while a nurse pumped air into my lungs with an ambu bag.

In Hebrews 13:5 the Bible (KJV) quotes God as saying to His children, "I will never leave thee, nor forsake thee." In the dark night of my ordeal, it sometimes *seemed* as though He had deserted me. But then someone would do something or say something that would reassure me that, in spite of all the clouds, the sun was still shining, God was still sovereign, and that this trial would pass.

"[God] doesn't treat us as our sins deserve, nor pay us back in full for our wrongs. As high as heaven is over the earth, so strong is his love to those who fear him. And as far as sunrise is from sunset, he has separated us from our sins. As parents feel for their children, God feels for those who fear him." — Psalm 103:10-13, *The Message*

During his stay and afterward, I have come to understand and appreciate this man of the cloth. What the psychiatrist described as "rough and mean" I see as this man's initial, desperate and frightened attempt at regaining some semblance of control in his life. As Daryl later wrote, *This was a terrible time of testing, and my courage faltered badly . . . At times a crisis may crack so suddenly, so closely, and so violently that we will impulsively react in some inappropriate way, causing us to feel even worse about ourselves.* In his efforts to help others in similar circumstances, Daryl further wrote that *[the] challenge is to live May in March, to believe in the sun even when it isn't shining.* He also offered that sometimes the only thing that comes closest to helping in such challenging circumstances is *just quiet, human companionship. The sort of companionship that does not make an attempt to offer easy answers or quick cures for deep hurt; companionship that does not try to handily diagnose the cause of the suffering; companionship that in no way condemns; companionship that just offers a steady, consistent, unconditional, quiet concern and presence; companionship that is sensitive and readily available.*

On a serene summer day many years later in 2011, I invited Daryl to speak at a little church in the small coastal town of South Addison. Though he and the pastor had not coordinated the readings and his message beforehand, they fit together perfectly. Both centered around suffering, and when Daryl saw my wife and me in the pews toward the end of his sermon, he began to get choked up. The experience was still fresh in his mind.

In the ICU we never felt he was either "rough" or "mean;" I'm not sure why things seemed to fall apart when he was transferred. Despite the medical center's policy discouraging relationships with former or current patients, I came to love this man as a friend and to admire his work and words of wisdom from the pulpit. Ultimately, he became the only patient with whom I ever remained in contact. I held him in such high esteem, in fact, that I could think of no one better suited to preside over my young daughter Jane's funeral in 2007. Every year on the anniversary of her death, I listen to the recorded words he spoke that day, words that lifted me from my sorrow though I could not lift Reverend Daryl from his wheelchair. "It's hard to understand why," he gently began.

> "Birds sing after a storm; why shouldn't people feel as free to delight in whatever sunlight remains to them?"
> ~Rose Kennedy, mother of President John F. Kennedy

Chapter 7: The Funny Pages/Moments of Insanity

T he American Heritage Dictionary defines *comic relief* as "a humorous or farcical interlude in a serious literary work or drama, especially a tragedy, intended to relieve the dramatic tension or heighten the emotional impact by means of contrast." We as nurses are caught up in the often twisted and tragic details of life and death every day and thus require comic relief in order to remain sane. Interjecting bits of humor along the sometimes painful and thorny path provides an outlet by which we can relieve some of the tension. As promised in the foreword, some of the following represent entertaining snapshots of such moments; others are humorous moments nurses and others would appreciate.

Patients whose capacity for understanding is compromised or limited---as is often the case with pediatric, mentally challenged, brain-injured, or memory-loss patients---present special needs that must be met before trust can be won. Discovering what these needs are is critical to their care. As an illustration, one of our excellent speech pathologists, Lorraine, once held a group therapy session with patients who all suffered from hemispatial neglect secondary to stroke. This means that if they'd sustained damage to the right hemispheres of their brains and were asked to fill in the face of a blank clock, there would be no numbers entered from 6:00 to 12:00. Lorraine provided a lunch for them at a round table. When she entered the dining area, she was surprised to see all of the patients eating out of the plates of the persons sitting to their right.

Kelly was a sweet, middle-aged woman with a genetic condition known as *Down syndrome.* Down syndrome results in varying degrees of physical and mental disability. Her constant companion was a stuffed bear she called "Teddy." Other than Teddy and the medical staff, she had no close relatives or friends who came to visit, no one with whom she could confide or consult.

We decided to enlist Teddy's help. When she needed an X-ray, Teddy also needed to go to X-ray. We passed one of our veteran radiology techs, Ed, on our way into the radiology department not long after Kelly's admission. He was reading an X-ray and shaking his head.

"What's up?" I asked, wheeling Kelly and Teddy around the room with the flair of a bellhop wheeling in room service.

Ed showed me the X-ray. I recognized a set of lungs dotted with a few small white, disc-shaped silhouettes.

"This is a negative of my chest."

I flinched, and my brows knit an unspoken question as I looked at my colleague in horror.

"Don't ever try to stifle a sneeze with a handful of thumbtacks," he said, still shaking his head. "The experts must have known about this hazard when they advised people to sneeze into their elbows." Poor Ed. Just the previous week, the wheel of his X-ray cart had caught a supporting post in the glass window that formed one whole wall of Room 142 in ICU, causing it to suddenly shatter and come crashing down.

I looked at Kelly and smiled. She was laughing and showing Teddy the X-ray.

After visiting radiology, Kelly's physician decided a CT scan might be helpful, and I wheeled the pair to the next building. A man lay on the gurney ahead of us while a huddle of healthcare professionals and family members surrounded a brightly lit screen. Radiologist Jill beckoned me to come see what they were discussing.

"I'll be right back," I said to Kelly and Teddy, who both smiled back at me.

"What's up?" I asked, reaching Jill just as she turned in the direction of the screen.

"Look at the image on the screen. What does it look like to you?"

I studied the image of a head scan for just a few seconds, as it resembled closely just one thing to me.

"Looks just like the head of a buffalo, like the ones on old nickels."

In unison, the huddled mass of bewildered radiologists, physicians, and family members turned around and nodded at me.

"Exactly," Jill said. "This guy's a Native American from Indian Island. Came in with a head bleed after being struck by a car. His Penobscot Tribal name is 'Buffalo.'"

Kelly's CT scan was unremarkable compared to Buffalo's, and Teddy's, though we had to go on faith rather than hard evidence, did not have an image that resembled his namesake, Teddy Roosevelt. Kelly seemed very relaxed through it all, and we returned unscathed to the ICU. Afterward, when Kelly needed to go to the bathroom, so did Teddy. Teddy got IV's, EKG pads, and Band-Aids following phlebotomy. These things seemed to help our patient with testing that was unfamiliar and frightening to her. Teddy, after all, did not seem to mind the procedures. Beyond this, I was also careful to remember to ask if there was anything I could do for Kelly or Teddy before each procedure, as meeting an unrecognized basic need (such as providing a warm blanket or a trip to the bathroom) often puts patients at ease for the procedure.

Over the following weeks, as Kelly's condition deteriorated, Teddy continued to bring her comfort. Following Kelly's death, as was customary in those early days, I wrapped her jaw closed with gauze. The wrap started at the top of her head, passed securely around her jaw, and ran up the other side of her head to its starting place at the top of her head, where it was then tied off.

While doing the remaining post-mortem care, I asked Nurse Jason and Nurse Janet, two of Kelly's other caregivers, to come into her room. It was a sad death for all of us involved. What they found was so unexpected and touching that it resulted in a release of emotions from both nurses. Teddy, Kelly's friend and mentor, who had provided an open channel of trust between Kelly and the medical staff, lay next to his charge in one final selfless act, mimicking her lifeless body. Kelly's arm encircled Teddy's body, and Teddy's jaw was wrapped in the gauze---just like Kelly's. We knew Kelly would be smiling too.

"Once your brain becomes a pickle, it can't go back to being a cucumber."
~Barbara Krantz, doctor

Nurse Eileen was a veteran nurse, but some things still caught her by surprise. It was during one of those very cold Maine winter days, when the wind and snow were blowing in from the southwest, that Jerry came to the alcohol rehabilitation unit. Nurse Eileen picked up the brown paper bag in which his clothes and shoes had been packed by the emergency room nurses and held it at arm's length, trying to avoid the stench of sweat, dirt, and alcohol rising from it. She put it in the cupboard, locked the cupboard door, and turned to introduce herself.

"Hi, I'm Eileen. I'm going to be your nurse today. And I'm going to try to help you out as much as I can."

"Jerry--nice to meet you," he said with his hand outstretched.

Eileen was pleasantly surprised by Jerry's calm demeanor. She shook his hand and smiled, then went about the routine of orienting him to his surroundings and schedule. He listened intently as she explained how and when to use the call bell, how to control the lights near the bed, and how to adjust the bed controls. Nurse Eileen then explained policies such as the no smoking policy and the policy prohibiting contraband, and she told him he should not get out of bed without calling first for assistance. They then discussed Jerry's schedule, which would include group therapy meetings and visits from his physician. Eileen felt quite confident she'd answered Jerry's concerns and questions.

By suppertime, Jerry seemed quite comfortable and settled into the routine he would be following for the next few weeks. When the end of her shift came, Eileen bid her new patient a good night, wrote the name of the night shift nurse on a Post-it note, and tacked it to the bulletin board at the foot of his bed.

"Good night," he answered with a smile, his eyes twinkling. "Drive careful in this mess."

The next morning, Eileen was confronted on her way into Jerry's room by one of the security guards.

"Your patient enjoyed quite the night," he began.

"What?" Eileen opened the door wider and peeked into the room. Jerry appeared to be asleep in the same bed where she'd left him. "What do you mean?"

"It seems Jerry escaped in his johnny last night, found his way to his car, where he had clothes and money, and met up with his buddies at the local tavern. The watchman on duty last night caught him coming back through the main entrance, and when he questioned Jerry, well, Jerry was bombed out of his freakin' mind!"

Eileen looked in astonishment at Jerry, then at the watchman, then back at her patient. Did she dream yesterday, or was this yet another instance of a patient leaving the hospital against medical advice? The hospital certainly had seen its share of such instances. One of her patients on a 2.0 mg/minute lidocaine drip had ripped out his IV, run down the hall to the front door naked, and was never seen again. (So much for weaning his drip!) Not long afterward, another man wanted out after having endured open-heart surgery. He walked home a few streets down from the hospital in his johnny and with his pacing wires still in place. Only when one of the cardiac surgeons called and begged him to return did we finally get him back.

And how could she forget the construction worker who'd been impaled with rebar before OSHA's requirement of rebar caps? Initially, the family nicknamed the man "Spike," but once the rebar was in place for two weeks, Spike became "Rusty." After leaving the ICU and going to the fifth floor, Rusty jumped from the window to his death on the rocks below. The family sued for wrongful death, but the judge ruled that once this man left the window ledge, he effectively left AMA.

Still, this one would be a surprise to Eileen. Upon examination of her patient, it was obvious he was hung over, indeed confirming what the watchman had said.

During the last quarter of the twentieth century, the ICU experienced a seventy-five percent turnover rate of nursing staff. Our department manager, frustrated and unhappy, felt the source of the problem was an incompetent and insecure nursing pool, and she even resorted to having a psychiatrist come in to intervene. Our complaints of hard work with limited staffing and increased patient acuity seemed to fall on deaf ears. No one seemed to understand that patients—often lacking money for preventative care---were coming to the hospital sicker. Greater longevity was also ushering in patients much older and with more complicated comorbidities than ever before. Far from being sympathetic with the nurses, the department manager claimed a monkey could do their jobs better. Nurse Dawn B, indignant about having been singled out, didn't let us forget about it; it became our newest rallying cry.

To this day, when we need to compliment one of our staff, nothing says it quite as well. When a nurse participates in a successful code or a doctor gets a central line inserted after three previous physicians have failed, we like to let the person know he or she is "smarter than a monkey."

There came a time early in the twenty-first century when, having seen our former boss to her retirement, we needed to "orient" a new nurse manager and many other new staff nurses to the ICU. It happened to be a period during which we noticed a startling increase in the incidence of self-extubations (SE). An SE is the act of a patient prematurely pulling out his endotube. This tube is externally tied around the neck with a strap, and a balloon is inflated into the trachea to hold it in its internal position. Ninety percent of intubated patients (patients with breathing tubes inserted) wore restraints to keep them from accidentally or intentionally pulling out the endotubes. A restraint is a piece of cloth tied around the wrist and attached to a long strap tied to an anchor on the bedframe under the mattress. I was asked to figure out why the incidence of SEs was increasing.

Upon making my morning rounds, I noticed that many of the patients who were restrained had the long restraint strap tied under the mattress near the foot of the bed rather than near the hip area, and every patient who self-extubated had the restraint strap tied near the foot of the bed. It seemed intuitive that the patient could wiggle down in the bed and have plenty of slack to pull out the tube. My nurse manager Sue W seemed skeptical and didn't seem to quite grasp the concept. After several weeks and more extubation incidences, and seeing no apparent move toward educating the staff on proper restraint technique, I suggested to Sue it was time for a little "show-and-tell."

I asked Sue to come into an empty room and lie on the bed. I put a pair of restraints on her wrists and tied them to the foot of the bed.

"Wiggle down and scratch your nose," I directed.

This she did with ease. I then asked her to lie back down, and I retied the restraints to the anchor beneath her hip area.

"Now, pick your nose," I instructed her.

"I see what you mean," Sue conceded, unable to find enough slack in the strap to move very far.

Hours later, several other nurses asked if they could be next. I smiled at the thought . . . and in the self-satisfaction that maybe I was, after all, "smarter than a monkey."

"Trust in Allah, but tie your camel."
~Old Muslim Proverb

Nurse Beverly, Nurse Darla, and I were lucky enough one year to win the lottery held to send nurses to the American Association of Critical-Care Nurses National Teaching Institute convention. This one was being held in Las Vegas.

"Ray," Beverly said one day. "I just made the arrangements for our trip, and we had enough to cover one room for the three of us. May I ask you a favor?"

"Okay, Beverly," I said, anticipating what was coming. "Just remember that I'm a happily married man."

"The room has two beds. Darla doesn't want to sleep in my bed because I'm a lesbian. May I sleep with you in the other bed?"

I laughed at the situation and told her not to worry about it. We'd work something out.

Later that evening, I told my wife about the situation. Karen knew Beverly and me very well and knew we would never betray her. She laughed and said, "You'll work something out."

Flying into Las Vegas, I was struck with the isolation of this fun town. In its heart, Las Vegas was packed with the expected brightly lit neon signs of gambling casinos and entertainment establishments. Houses crowded its perimeter. Beyond the houses lay desert, miles and miles of sand.

Having never been to the Casino City before, I was anxious to try my hand at some of the games. Beverly was a veteran gambler, who knew the city well. Darla, well, Darla just came for the buffets.

It was 9:15 pm when we finally arrived in our hotel room, way past my bedtime. But this was a time when Beverly was accustomed to going out. Darla staked out her bed, piling her belongings on top of it. Beverly and I looked at each other and put our belongings on the floor in separate corners of the room. *We'll figure something out,* I thought, trying not to worry.

I donned my pajamas, brushed my teeth, and stepped out of the bathroom just in time to see Beverly step out the room door.

"See you tomorrow morning, "she said. "The night is young."

Seizing the opportunity while I could, I slipped into the unclaimed bed and off into La-La Land. Darla did the same on the other side of the room.

Beverly returned just as I was getting ready to go out, and she took my place in the bed after giving me a few pointers about gambling. I had passed up an invitation to go to breakfast and lunch with Darla, preferring instead to sleep.

And so it went. Beverly and I worked it out by rotating use of the bed and the gaming facilities. When the conference program began, Beverly took the 2:00 am to 2:00 pm gaming/meeting schedule, and I took the 2:00 pm to 2:00 am gaming/meeting schedule. Darla was not happy that she was forced to go alone to each meal.

"I have found out that there ain't no surer way to find out whether you like people or hate them than to travel with them."
~Mark Twain, author

"There ain't much fun in medicine, but there's a heck of a
lot of medicine in fun!"
~Josh Billings, humorist

Every year on April the 1ˢᵗ, a bogus version of our hospital newsletter,
Currents, would circulate. We suspected the perpetrator to be none
other than our resident comedian, Dr. T, and he did later admit
complicity. But the year after Dr. T died, the version mysteriously
materialized again, and we knew more jokers abounded to trap fools. In
fact, the 1982 issue advertised for more help, since "outwitting
Administration, though easy," would take some time and effort.

At first glance, the newsletter seemed legitimate. It was complete
with the hospital logo, printed on official, brightly-colored paper stock,
and included the telephone numbers of administrators as editors. Its
stories sent shock waves through the pool of loyal employees of the
healthcare facility and caught unseasoned readers off guard. There were
accounts of telephone operators being sent out to New York City to
receive additional training because a warm and friendly approach was
deemed "not suitable for a major medical center;" the offer to female
employees of free Advanced Bosom Scans with Computerized
Appendicular Mammography (ABSCAM) by the chief of radiology, who
was known to have a special interest in this area and who indicated he
would "personally inspect each case;" and a report of a marked increase
in the number of obscene phone calls received on the physician's
dictation system. Regarding the latter, the transcriptionists were
reportedly "handling the four-letter words pretty well but were having
trouble spelling the heavy breathing."

The 1980 issue of the newsletter came complete with a sample of a
new employee opinion poll suggested by the hospital CEO to give a
more accurate reflection of employee attitudes. It went something like
this:

Question	Response (Check one)		
	Very Good	Excellent	Superb
My salary is..................	_____	_____	_____
My hours are...............	_____	_____	_____
My supervisor is..........	_____	_____	_____
My prospects for advancement are...	_____	_____	_____

Other April 1 issues of *Currents* reported on an innovative new program for community leaders in which a new subsidiary of the hospital system would be able to sue our own system before outside attorneys got the chance, thereby improving upon our past record of Bangor lagging the nation in successful malpractice suits due to robust patient satisfaction with physician services; a new pitch to Maine's heretofore unresponsive Christian Science community, with an emphasis on non-healthcare related activities; the opening of a new, all-natural colonic lavage center at the old Waterworks Building just upstream from the hospital, which would utilize a special lift to lower patients into the healing waters of the Penobscot River, thereby flushing all impure matter from the colon and impure thoughts from the mind; the celebration of the current CEO's newest wing to the hospital as the "greatest erection of his career;" and the introduction of coin-operated wheelchairs.

In line with such antics on April 1, Secretary Pam thought she would have some fun with Dr. B, the Filipino physician with broken English who often mixed up his pronoun genders. Sadly, he had declared one of his patients brain dead in Room 147, and we were keeping the man's body there pending the family's visit the next day. Dr. B always took his patients' deaths to heart, and this one was no different.

He'd gone out of his way to pull strings and keep him in the room overnight.

The next morning, when Pam came into work, she dialed Dr. B's telephone number at home.

"Hi, Dr. B. It's Pam."

"Hello, Baby. What's up?"

"Sorry to bother you, but I need to tell you that your patient in Room 147 signed himself out AMA this morning."

There was silence on the other end.

"Dr. B?"

"Holy sheet! I thought . . . she'd was fooking dead . . . Holy sheet!"

It took a long time for Dr. B to understand this was only a joke, a carefully crafted prank sanctioned only on April 1. To this day, he makes doubly certain of his pronouncements.

The people Down East are some of the friendliest and most down-to-earth folk you'd ever want to meet. They are, in fact, one of the reasons why my wife and I recently relocated to the Down East area. We consider the town of South Addison, with its eighty or so residents, a kind of second family, and we've shared many stories about Down Easters.

From the beginning, my new neighbors made me feel at ease. My wife and I had been taking daily walks to the town landing and back, a round trip of about four miles, when my neighbor Oscar saw us start out one day and stopped us.

"You wouldn't want to take Beau here with you, would you?"

I looked down at Beau, a beautiful reddish-brown Boykin spaniel, who was beginning to jump about with the frenzied excitement that visitors in his yard spawned.

"Well, Oscar," I began. Oscar had always been straightforward with me, and I reciprocated. It was a great relationship. "I wouldn't mind, but there's something disgusting about picking up warm poop in a plastic bag."

Oscar looked at me incredulously, his mouth drawn up in a circle and his head tilted to one side. "Ray," he said, "this is South Addison. We don't do such a thing here. They'd think you was stealin' it!"

Just a hop, skip, and a jump away from South Addison is the small town of Milbridge. Kenney, a nurse who hailed from Milbridge, had probably the thickest Down East accent and the driest sense of humor I'd ever encountered. He was also not the crispiest cucumber in the salad. One of his patient assignments at a hospital across town from our medical center necessitated the use of Dopamine, a very powerful IV drug commonly used in critical care settings to increase blood pressure. Dopamine is usually dripped in and is reported in micrograms per kilogram per minute. The range usually employed is anywhere from 2.0 to 20.0 micrograms per kilo per minute. When the administered dose approaches 20 micrograms per kilo per minute, most physicians switch the patient to another vasoactive drug to avoid complications and ensure success.

"How much Dopamine is she on?" asked Dr. O, upon making his rounds.

"She's lovin' all the Dopamine I can give 'er," answered Kenney in his thick accent.

"How much?"

"She's lovin' all the Dopamine I can give 'er," he repeated more loudly, stone-faced.

Kenney mysteriously left employment at this hospital soon after the incident.

Two weeks later, Dr. O made his debut rounds at our hospital's ICU. I was in the nursing station viewing a patient chart when he came into the unit, sat down with a cup of coffee, and also began reviewing a patient chart. Not long afterward, he got up to answer a phone call. Nurses have a way of sizing things up rather quickly, and as Dr. O looked harmless enough, I thought I would have a little fun to welcome him to our hospital.

When he sat back down, I pushed his coffee cup closer to him. "Next time, put a little more cream in it, Doc," I said.

Out of the corner of my eye, I watched as Dr. O picked up the cup. He didn't laugh; he didn't look angry. He just took a sip of his coffee. I had a sinking feeling he didn't have a sense of humor after all. *Oh, rats.*

In a monotone, he said, "Well, you didn't have to pee in it."

I knew we'd get along splendidly.

A few moments later, Dr. O walked into Room 137 and, while looking down at the chart, asked the attending nurse how much Dopamine the patient was getting.

"He's lovin' all the Dopamine I can give 'im," came the reply.

Dr. O slowly raised his head and stared at a smiling Kenney, whose successful transfer had landed him squarely back with Dr. O.

"You don't have to hear it, but you should be able to recite it."
~ Dean Harrison, RN, BSN

Nurse Barbara was working the night shift on the neurology unit and had just given a dose of morphine to one of her new admissions, Cathy. She settled down at the nursing station for a quick cup of coffee while reviewing charts, when Cathy rang her on the intercom.

"Yes," Barbara said. "What can I do for you?"

"There's a big rat under my bed!" came the excited cry.

Barbara looked at her coworker, who raised her eyebrows. "I'll be right there," she promised, retrieving the flashlight from the power emergency drawer.

As Barbara walked down the long corridor to Cathy's room at the end, she thought about some of the stories she'd heard about rodents in the building. Unwelcome pests had at one time been a problem in the lab and in ICU on the first floor, some thought because of the hospital's proximity to the Penobscot River. Still, this was the fifth floor, pest issues had long ago been resolved, and she had, after all, just given a *neuro* patient a dose of morphine, a drug whose name is derived from Morpheus, the Greek god of sleep and dreams.

Barbara was an exceptionally kind and gentle nurse. She knew the majority of nurses would probably have dismissed the rat sighting as a hallucination secondary to the morphine. She remembered the fall day when Nurse Michelle had given her trauma patient 50 mcg of Fentanyl, only to have the patient ring her twenty minutes later with a report of bees in the room. In the chart, Michelle had noted the next dose of Fentanyl should be decreased, and a superficial check of the room put the patient's mind at ease. A few hours later, though, the room was swarming with the insects. There was a nest just outside the window, and they'd found a convenient escape from the coming winter through a hole in the screen of the slightly open window.

Barbara glanced into Room 523 as she walked by and reassured herself that her other patient was sleeping soundly. She had erred on the side of *this* patient earlier in the day, and the incident was still fresh in her mind.

"Do you wear glasses?" she had asked the new patient in 523.

"Yes, but I forgot to bring them."

"Would you like me to see if one of your family members can bring them in?"

"No, I need them only for reading."

Barbara had watched as the new admission fumbled with picking up drinking cups and eating utensils. Not satisfied the patient was being one hundred percent truthful about needing her glasses, she retrieved the most colorful johnny she could find from the freshly washed linens. It was somewhere between a bright lime green and a neon yellow, with royal blue drawstring ties.

"Look at this johnny I found for you. Aren't these ties a bright color?"

"I can't see them," the patient confessed.

Barbara realized she'd been too trusting.

She was starting to blame herself for giving Cathy too much morphine, when she reached her room and found her scrunched up under the covers in the middle of the bed. Barbara shone the light under the bed.

"It's not there anymore," she said, convinced now there was no rat.

"He ran under the heater!" the patient yelled from under her covers.

Barbara obligingly went through the motions of looking under the heater with her flashlight. To her great surprise, the unmistakable bright yellow glint of two eyes shone back at her.

When the varmint was at last captured under an empty gauze box, it was determined to be not a rat, but a gerbil---an escapee from the children's ward a full two buildings away. "Oh, rats," the rest of us moaned, cringing at the thought there would still be a rodent on the loose, if one of *us* had been assigned this patient.

When I was a coffee drinker, I often got myself a cup in the ICU's little kitchen during my morning or afternoon break. One morning I could find no packaged cream or containers of milk in the staff refrigerator or cupboard, but I did see a few Styrofoam cups with lids in the refrigerator. Each of these were about three quarters full of milk, and I helped myself to one of them, appreciative someone had apparently taken the time to make more room for staff lunches by getting rid of the larger containers.

On her way home that afternoon, Nurse Mary bumped into me having another cup in the kitchen, and shaking her head with discontent, she commented, "I could've sworn I pumped more than this today." She picked up a mason jar of milk and a Styrofoam cup from the refrigerator, showed it to me, and placed it in her insulated bag for the trip home for her new baby. She was one of three new mom nurses in the unit. "I'm just going to have to drink more, so I can produce more," she shrugged. I looked up and smiled at her, painfully aware of my error.

My mind's eye drifted off to the baby shower I'd attended several months earlier . . .

. . . I'd filled a baby bottle with Maalox, labeled it "Propofol," and gave it to Mary. "This is 'Mommy's little helper,'" I'd joked. (Propofol is a white liquid given in IV form to a patient who needs to be immediately sedated.)

It seemed harmless enough, especially considering how much Mary loved a good laugh. She and her husband Mike had wanted a baby for years, but not until Mike was deployed by the military and overseas for a month did she discover they were expecting. She freely shared with us details of the day she was to have her first gynecologic exam after taking the pregnancy test. It was the third of July, and Mary had offered to watch her niece at her home while Mary's sister ran a few errands.

"I'll be back in time for you to get to your appointment," her sister promised.

Mary spent a fun-filled morning with her niece making decorations for the Fourth, and she hardly noticed the time ticking by. Thirty minutes prior to her scheduled appointment time, however, Mary started to panic. It was at least a fifteen-minute drive to her doctor's—under the best conditions—and she still needed to shower.

"Made it!" her sister said, bursting through the door. She scooped up her daughter, and they headed out, thanking Mary and wishing her luck at the doctor's.

There was no time for a shower. Mary grabbed a washcloth hanging near the sink and gave herself a sponge bath. "I'm my own patient today," she said, chuckling and thinking of the many times she'd bathed a patient this way.

Sitting down in her doctor's waiting room, Mary practiced a little slow breathing to reduce her blood pressure, which she assumed would be elevated with all the scurrying about she'd done. She felt pretty relaxed by the time she put her legs up in the stirrups.

"Wow, happy Fourth of July to you too!" the doctor said to Mary during the exam.

Mary was confused but didn't want her doctor to think she hadn't wished him a happy holiday. She smiled in silence. He removed his gloves, said all was well, made a note on her chart, and asked her to set up an appointment for September.

When Mary returned home later that afternoon, she noticed that the washcloth she'd used for her sponge bath was covered in red, white, and blue glitter and remembered her niece had used the bathroom to wash up. She made a mental note to explain the glitter to her gynecologist in September.

The rest of Mary's pregnancy was uneventful, and when Mike's tour of duty ended ten months later, he was very excited to be able to see his new son for the first time. Mary left the baby in the care of her mother and went to the crowded airport to meet his plane. When they arrived home, Mary's mother met them at the door and told them the baby was asleep in his baby carriage. They tiptoed to the carriage, and Mary gently uncovered the sleeping baby so that Mike could see him.

"Arrgh!" he cried, jumping back.

Mike's son was covered in a coat of brown fur. To Mike's shock, Mary had substituted a live chimpanzee (borrowed from a neighbor) for his son, who was really asleep in his crib upstairs . . .

. . . I later admitted to Nurse Mary that I'd accidentally fallen victim to an unintentional booby trap and had drunk her breast milk.

"No sense crying over spilled milk," she said, smiling too broadly.

"I'm sorry," I stammered. "It didn't taste quite right, but--you know, maybe we should institute our labeling rules."

"I'll help you stay abreast of any updates about that," Mary replied.

That night I slept like a baby, but, having been busted, I was harassed for years and even accused of "milking situations for all they were worth." I was given stationery with the heading "Lactation Consultant" from the OB/GYN floor and was told I was so young-looking that I still had mother's milk on my lips. Actually, it was the first winter in a long time in which I didn't get a cold.

Room 148 was directly opposite the entrance to the waiting room. In fact, there was no avoiding it when visitors came to the coronary care unit just beyond. It was the only room available one morning when Randy was admitted. Gray-haired Randy, 87 years young, was a streaker. Every chance he got, he took off his clothes. Redressing him and putting him back to bed became routine. Because he was persistently getting out of bed, we also needed to keep the curtains to his room pulled open.

Not long after Randy was admitted, we got word our accrediting agency, the Joint Commission on Accreditation of Healthcare Organizations (JACHO), was scheduled to make a stop in the unit. Everything was in place. There'd been only one minor incident that morning, when Nurse Lori had come running to me from the break room with word the toaster was on fire. She'd left it on high and had been sidetracked with a patient emergency, when she saw smoke coming from that direction. Luckily, I was able to pick up the burning appliance with a couple of wet towels and toss it out the window and into a snowbank, before the smoke alarm sounded and fire trucks were dispatched. We had three minutes to spare before D-Day.

As I stood at the main desk in the ICU, I could see the inspectors rounding the corner to enter our unit. I looked in the opposite direction, and there was old Randy in all his glory, his johnny pulled up high over his head. "Nurse Joan," I said hurriedly. "There's a gray squirrel in 148."

Peter Jennings once said that the best sight is hindsight. This never rang truer to me than when Steve came into our unit. He'd been in a horrific motorcycle crash, and his girlfriend Becky stayed faithfully by his side twenty-four-seven.

It wasn't long before we noticed a definite disdain Becky seemed to have for someone named "Mary." There were cards found in the wastebasket signed by Mary, and there were phone calls from Mary, which mysteriously got disconnected.

"Who is 'Mary?'" one nurse asked Becky a week after Steve was admitted.

If glares came equipped with claws, that nurse would not be among the living. She quickly backed down and never mentioned Mary again.

Not long afterward, Steve was well enough to be bathed from head to toe. It was then that the nurse bathing him was able to make out and finally read a remarkable tattoo on the underside of the young motorcyclist's manhood. In small letters that we knew would expand greatly in font size and clout at the most inappropriate of times were the words, "Promised to Mary."

Later, when Steve's young son visited, we looked at each other with the shared secret hope that he didn't have a tattoo on *his* kickstand.

"The difference between love and regrets is that regrets last forever."
~Drew Mosher-Buyno, age fourteen

"Two roads diverged in a wood, and I—I took the one less traveled by, and that has made all the difference."
~Robert Frost, poet

Charlene had worked as a nurse so long that we determined she'd probably changed some of our diapers in the obstetrics unit. She was working in the days when polio was rampant and iron lungs were in vogue. She was working when the rest of us were getting smallpox vaccinations. And she worked at a time when disposables were not yet in widespread use. Disposable gloves were rarely used and were reserved for high-risk exposure cases, and disposable isolation gowns were never seen outside of the OR. In those days, as we still do, Charlene laundered her own uniforms. (Only the OR staff used scrubs at that time.) She was meticulous and made sure she wore a freshly washed and starched, crisp white uniform each day she worked.

Charlene was part of a lovely little family, a husband and a sweet and affable daughter, Lynne, who was confined to a wheelchair. Because of her daughter's immobility and compromised state, Charlene was especially on the alert for anything contagious that might endanger her family's health. They made their home in a crowded urban neighborhood just a few miles from the hospital.

One night while covering a shift in the ICU, Charlene was assigned to care for Ben, a gentleman with a very debilitating and severe condition. The physicians were not sure what was causing his symptoms, and they cautioned the caregivers to wash their hands with soap and water when leaving his room (which was, of course, not yet standard practice). Charlene had seen a few of her friends succumb to illnesses they had contracted in the unit, and she was very careful to follow this suggestion.

"Good morning, Ben," she said, handing him his morning meds. "I'll be back again tonight." She washed her hands thoroughly, gave report, put on her coat, and left for the day.

The neighborhood was just gearing up for a rising sun when she arrived at her doorstep. She looked around and noticed lights coming on in the houses around her yard, and she imagined parents hauling reluctant children from their comfortable beds to get them ready to catch the school bus. They would be jealous of her being able to go to bed now. Not wanting to disturb her family, she clicked on the light just inside the door, which was a good distance from the bedrooms. Glancing out the window, she could see the Bentons reading the *Bangor Daily* at their kitchen table. It was a cozy little neighborhood.

On her ride home, Charlene had decided she would remove all of her clothes before venturing very far into her home. That way, she could throw all the possibly contaminated clothing into the washer, which was just inside the entry. The living room, which lay between the entry and the nearest bedroom, was still somewhat dark, and she decided it would be best to keep the entry light on to avoid tripping over anything. Looking again over at the Benton's, Charlene decided the safest way to do all of this was to get down on all fours---under window level. She certainly didn't want to be accused of exposing herself.

She removed her coat and shoes and put them off to the side. Then Charlene sat on the floor and removed her uniform, slip, underwear and pantyhose, slid the delicates into a small mesh bag, and did a kind of four-legged lay-up to the open washer.

There, she thought to herself. *I'll just wash my hands when I get to the bathroom, where I can stand up.*

Stealthily, she walked on her hands and knees to avoid being seen by neighbors in the partially lit rooms. When she neared the lower level of the picture window, she dropped onto her belly and crawled. Her husband always left a little light on for her in the kitchen, which lay off to one side of the living room, and she thought she could reach up high enough to flip the light off on her way by.

"Hellooo!" a voice exclaimed, as she raised her arm to reach the switch. Her husband didn't sound like himself. Startled, her eyes shot up and looked into the red face of her brother-in-law, who had arrived unexpectedly at the bus station a few blocks away late the previous night. He and Charlene's husband were enjoying a cup of coffee in the subdued light and were surprised by Charlene's quiet, but spectacular, entrance.

"Take time to deliberate, but when the time for action has arrived, stop thinking and go in."
~ Napoleon Bonaparte, military commander

"It's the second mouse that gets the cheese."
~ Sir Colin Spedding, biologist

Blood-sucking leeches have long been used medicinally following various reconstructive and plastic surgeries, including limb or appendage reattachment, in which there is often venous congestion due to inefficient drainage. The bloodletting, combined with the anticoagulant property of the leeches' saliva, reduces swelling and promotes healing by allowing fresh, oxygenated blood to reach the affected area.

We get the leeches for use in the ICU from the pharmacists, who in turn keep the little darlings content in a jar of fresh water until needed. A suitable number for the job (usually one or two) is applied to the affected area and is allowed to engorge for twenty minutes to two or more hours. When satiated, a leech drops off, plumped up and happy. We nurses like to name the leeches; it seems to allow for a friendlier leech/patient experience.

After one such surgery, Nurse Blaine applied a couple of leeches he had christened "Fred" and "Ethyl" to the reattached hand of a young woman who had been in a motorcycle crash. Ethyl got right down to business, but the sleeker, blacker male did a little head wave before chowing down. Blaine checked on the patient and, satisfied the leeches would not be a problem for her, left to check on his other patient.

It turned out to be a very busy afternoon. When Blaine returned an hour later to check on the leeches, they were already finished with their meal. Ethyl had dropped onto the sheets below the slightly elevated arm, but pesky Fred was nowhere to be found. Blaine plopped Ethyl into her water receptacle and scoured the bed linens and the area surrounding the bed for Fred. After several minutes of searching, he came upon a slimy trail. It led out the door and down the hall.

Trying to be inconspicuous, Blaine followed the trail. He bumped into Nurse Roland.

"Oh, sorry, Roland. Hey, if you were a leech, where would you hide?"

"Huh?" Roland asked.

Blaine smiled, waved his arms in dismissal, and moved on down the hall. The trail went past Room 147, then 148, then veered suddenly into the lunchroom.

As luck would have it, I had organized a potluck. Our potlucks were beyond compare, something nurses orienting to the department realized very early on. After having oriented Nurse Barbara earlier in the week, I asked her if she baked pies.

"Yes, I do," she responded.

"We're having a potluck on Sunday. Could you bring a pie?"

"Sure," she agreed.

Upon encountering other staff later that day, I told them Barbara was bringing a pie and asked if they could bring something as well so that we could have a potluck. Things had worked out splendidly.

"Hello, Blaine," the girls said cheerfully, as Blaine entered the lunchroom. He looked up in surprise and saw nurses, housekeepers, and receptionists sitting around the room, their plates filled with a colorful array of appetizers, relishes, sandwiches, and casseroles--- including their perennial favorite, tuna noodle casserole. Beyond them the table was overflowing with an assortment of pies, cookies, and squares.

"Grab some food," they encouraged, handing Blaine a plate.

Blaine looked around nervously. He glanced at the trail of slime, noticing with a sense of trepidation that it followed the table leg up to the feast. As he filled his plate, he continued to follow the trail. It ended at what must have seemed to Fred like a veritable Garden of Eden, an ornate little oasis filled with water and black olives. Blaine noticed Fred's characteristic head wave among the other black baubles and breathed a sigh of relief.

Pawing through the dish would not be good form, he thought, remembering how slippery the little rascals are. He scooped the whole dish of black olives into his plate. Some of the others noticed Blaine's love for olives but politely said nothing.

Now what? Blaine thought to himself. *I can't bring food out of the lunchroom, and I certainly don't want to eat Fred.*

Roland walked in then and surveyed the table. Roland was a Frenchman with a love for French dishes like frogs' legs and escargot. "No more olives?" he asked.

"Here, take mine." Blaine said. "I can't eat all these." He handed the plate to Roland and grabbed a cookie on the way out. "Bon appetit!" he said.

"Forgive, O Lord, my little jokes on Thee, And I'll forgive
Thy great big one on me."
~Robert Frost, poet, "Cluster of Faith," 1962

Things are not always as they might first appear. Two elderly ladies sat in the front of our hospital chapel during service one Sunday morning. The chaplain noticed that one of the ladies was talking during his sermon. He tried to remain calm and simply raised his voice a bit. As he did so, the lady also raised her voice. At the end of the sermon, the chaplain caught up with the pair and chastised the lady for being rude. As it turned out, the lady's friend was hearing-impaired and needed a louder voice in her ear to hear the sermon.

Chaplains are wise to avoid assumptions and to make sure those listening to their word can actually hear it. In the same way, compliance by end users of medical technology can become strained if the needs of the end users are not taken into account. I was always baffled, for instance, by the Blood Bank's insistence that we nurses---sometimes in the midst of saving a patient's life---identify and document each bag of blood with a number that was upside down and backwards (since the bag hung upside down from the way it was labeled). How simple it would be for Blood Bank technologists, who are free to handle, turn, place and read the bag label in any direction, to place the label so that it could be read right side up when hung at the bedside!

The laboratory also worked closely with some of the country's best biotech engineers, who kept the lab's equipment in top-notch condition.

Karen was a lab technologist, whose work required use of a fluorescent microscope.

"Hi, Dan," Karen said. "You installed a microscope bulb last week, and we're having trouble with it. The field of vision is half obliterated, so it seems the bulb needs to be centered better."

"No problem—I'll be over to align it with you when you and the scope are available."

Later that day, Karen and Dan turned the scope light on and the room lights off. They closed the door most of the way to keep extraneous light, which might quench the fluorescent dye used on the test slide, away from their work area. Centering the bulb required Karen to look into the oculars and report on what happened while Dan patiently turned the screws of the lamphouse clockwise or counterclockwise. The goal was to get the light to completely fill the field of vision, and painstakingly finding the right combination of each screw position was a challenge.

I happened to be in the lab and walking by the partially closed door, when I heard the following exchange:

"That's it—that's the spot . . . Oh, that's good . . . Uh, huh. That's good. . . A little lower . . . Yes . . . This feels so good [to have it finally working] . . . Oh, Dan, keep going, a little higher--that's the spot—that's so good! Yes . . . yes . . . yes!!!"

"Karen . . ."

Silence followed, as I surmised that an embarrassed Karen realized what her exclamations of joy must have sounded like. Things are not always as they might first appear.

If anyone can claim to have seen it all, especially in regards to body orifices, it's an emergency room doctor. People learn from an early age that body orifices need occasional cleaning out. What mother has never found her child picking his nose? The intriguing thing is that some people want to spice this up a little by filling a void and *expanding their horizons*, so to speak. They present with an assortment of articles in their other orifices: cucumbers, carrots, bananas (a veritable salad!); gerbils.

One of our gastroenterologists was called one evening to remove a vibrator from the rectum of a middle-aged man. Accompanying the patient to our unit afterward due to perforation of the bowel, the doctor commented to me, "I wasn't sure if he wanted me to change the battery or turn it off."

Working in the emergency room presented an intense, if not interesting, environment and challenged its workers to stay focused. Nurse Tina first arrived in Bangor as an emergency room nurse just as one of the first fast-food restaurants in the city—or for that matter, in the state—was also making its debut, and just as she was finding it difficult to juggle the demands of a household, a growing family, and a 7:00 am to 3:00 pm nursing shift. Nurse Velma bumped into her as Tina was hurrying out the door one sunny afternoon in early autumn.

"Oh, sorry," she said.

"My fault," Tina said, looking over her shoulder, then walking backwards away from Velma. "I've got a ton of errands to run before I pick up my kids."

"Try the new McDonald's—it'll save you from having to make supper." Velma's last words drifted into oblivion as Tina rounded the corner. Velma looked out the window and watched Tina run across the entrance and toward the parking lot.

Tina wondered if she had remembered to chart her last patient's vital signs.

By 4:00 pm Tina had stopped at Bangor Savings and cashed her check, after which she headed over to Doug's Shop'n Save to do the weekly grocery shopping. She studied the receipt and congratulated herself for having saved ten dollars compared to the previous week's food bill. *Maybe I can stop by that fast food joint after all*, she thought. *I called radiology about the head injured patient, didn't I?* She smiled a bit, as she mentally walked through the last ten minutes of her shift and saw herself dialing the number for radiology. *Of course, I did.*

By 4:40, Tina had picked up her children at the after-school program and at the babysitter's house. Her husband Joe was always home promptly at 5:00 pm, about the time she could be home with burgers and fries from McDonald's. *Why not? It'll be fun for a change.*

She turned into the newly tarred driveway under great golden arches and a large sign that announced the franchise's grand opening: "Two burgers for the price of one." Cheers arose from the backseat of her new 1964 Volvo, and she felt for the first time in a long time the jubilation of being able to "do it all."

Looking into the back seat, she made sure the children were still buckled in. "Sit tight. Mommy will be right back."

Tina got out of the car, locked the doors, and looked up at the new one-story building with a polished silver exterior. Inside she could see a line of patrons beginning to form. She'd overheard some of her coworkers discussing the convenience of ordering your food at a cute little window and being served almost immediately with hot food, packaged to go. It sounded too good to be true. *I'm glad Dr. H was on today. He's always so cheerful.*

Rounding the freshly planted hedges along the walkway, she noticed one of those little windows, and it was not currently being utilized by other customers. *It's my lucky day.*

"Hello," she began. She looked over at the outdoor menu board and confidently continued.

"I'd like to order four cheeseburgers, two vanilla shakes, two chocolate shakes, two small fries, and two large fries." *This is so easy—we'll have to come back if the food is good.*

Several groups of people walked past her as she was ordering, and she marveled at how convenient this all seemed for everyone. She was eager to get home and tell her husband about it. A lady stopped and smiled at her, then continued past her, looking for another window at which to order.

When two minutes passed, Tina's enthusiasm began to wane.

"Hello? Can you hear me?" she shouted into the window, now less than confident anyone was listening.

A tall man in a business suit, who had been sitting in his car across from Tina's window, got out of his car and strode toward her.

What a nice man! He'll get their attention for me.

"Excuse me, Ma'am," he began. "You can order inside or at the drive-through window on the other side."

"Oh, this one's *already* out of order, huh?"

"That's a wastebasket, Ma'am."

Tina stepped back, her mouth in a circle, and looked at the wastebasket she'd been talking into. She smiled at the teens walking past her with their fingers pointed toward her, then quietly walked back to her car and put the Volvo in reverse.

Some people have a natural or learned talent for remembering names. I, on the other hand, have always had a difficult time with it. Dr. H, recognizing this, taught me a neat little trick for overcoming this difficulty.

"Where I come from, African Americans always call each other by the nickname 'Jack' because they don't remember each other's names either."

From then on, I used his technique and called many people "Jack," but sometimes my reputation preceded me, especially when someone new was orienting to the department.

"Oh, once you've been around the unit for ten years, Ray will get your name right. But before then, don't count on it." This was one of the comments that was frequently bandied about, and I got kind of used to hearing it.

One sunny afternoon in early spring of the year I had semi-retired and joined the *pool*, one of the long-time nurses, Karyn C, gave me a hug and a compliment after I helped her locate some charts.

"Ray, you are amazing," she began. "You work here just twenty days out of the year, and yet you can make decisions and solve problems as if you were still here every day."

"Why, thank you," I said, feeling my head puff up a bit. "Funny, there's a nurse I haven't seen for a long while," I commented, running my fingers over the schedule from top to bottom. "She hasn't been on the schedule either. I wonder whatever happened to her."

"What's her name, Ray?"

"Her name was Karen," I said, scratching my head.

"Karen Who?"

I tried to access the appropriate interface in my brain with my cerebral flash drive and began to envision all of the Karens I knew. I thought about my sweet wife, whose name was Karen. But this Karen was one of my coworkers. She always impressed me as very professional in her demeanor and also in her dress. A clean, short lab coat distinguished her from the rest of us, and there was never a word or a hair out of place. I tried to associate her name with one of her characteristics, a technique which was suggested to me by one of my other colleagues. The most striking thing about Karen was her mascara. It was dark and matched her black hair. Did she transfer to another unit within the hospital? Did she and her husband of thirty years follow her daughter, who had moved to Florida—land of the infamous hanging chads? *Bingo!*

"Her name was Karyn Chadbourne," I said with confidence.

"Ray, *I* am Karyn Chadbourne," Karyn said without batting an accepting eyelash.

Hoping my nemesis, name amnesia, hadn't cancelled out all the praise Karyn had just heaped upon me, I laughed and said, "Oh, I'm sorry. I meant Karen Boudreau."

Richard, RN, who worked in the ER, was unlucky enough to have been born at a time when his nickname, "Dick," had a second meaning. I'd had enough of a hard time with my own middle name of "Peter" growing up, but "Dick" was worse, and I vowed never to have a "Dick" for a kid.

Dick was the favorite target of one particular and pompous nurse anesthetist, Nurse Gerald, who often used clever but biting words when conversing with his coworkers. Gerald was once admitted for a bowel obstruction. Because he felt no other nurse was capable of inserting a nasal gastric tube properly, cocky Gerald put it in himself.

Gerald usually saw Dick during codes, when nurse anesthetists were needed in the ER to intubate the patients. During the highly charged environment of a code, when the patient's room was crowded with many personnel—doctors; nurses; lab, X-ray and EKG technicians; respiratory therapists; and observers—it wasn't uncommon to hear Gerald ask Richard, "Got any gum on ya Dick?" Since no one ever rewarded him with a laugh, he eventually dropped this performance.

Perhaps due to the ribbing he got, Dick learned to be very clever with his own words. He would often go to the cafeteria, survey the choices, which might include mashed potatoes, chicken breast, green

240

beans, and freshly baked yeast rolls, and say to one of the women who stood behind the steaming food warmers, "I'll have one of your breasts."

One thing Dick was very proud of was his truck. He'd saved up all of his money and bought a Victory Red Chevy Silverado SS, equipped with a 6.0-liter Vortec High-Output V8 rated at 345 horsepower at 5200 rpm and 380 lb-ft of torque at 4000 rpm coupled to a 4L60E four-speed automatic transmission. The all-wheel drive setup also came with Z60 performance suspension and 20-inch aluminum wheels. A real beauty.

Dick treated his truck with white kid gloves, washing and waxing it religiously. No one was ever allowed to eat in the truck, and instead of wearing out the blinkers, Dick went back to the old system of hand signals. Years later, when the truck died at the very respectable age of 200,000 miles, AAA came and towed it to the junkyard at the edge of town. The only things still working on it were the blinkers.

One fall day just prior to his truck's demise, Dick got into trouble when the fallen, wet leaves made driving slick. His Silverado swerved out of control and struck a guardrail. Though his injuries were non-life-threatening, a piece of metal from the cab of his truck damaged the femoral artery in his left groin, and he spent a few days in the ICU recuperating from the excessive blood loss. One of the drugs he was given was Dopamine, a substance pharmacologic logic predicted would increase his blood pressure. Nursing Supervisor Harriet, whom we loved dearly, brought Dick in a *Playboy* magazine, which he hid under his butt. A few days later, she asked me how Dick was doing.

"Funniest thing," I said. "I've never seen a patient get weaned off his Dopamine so quickly."

When a patient has a low blood sodium level (*hyponatremia*), a doctor may write an order of "no free water." Seasoned caregivers know this means the patient should not have any extra water to drink. Such patients would derive all their water needs from the foods they ingest. Decreasing the water intake while maintaining dietary sodium at its present level has the net effect of increasing the *concentration* of blood sodium levels.

One of our new unit secretaries, Chloe, saw such an order and asked me how to enter it into the computerized billing system. That was like a mouse asking a cat to open its mouth.

"Well," I began. "Orders for 'no free water' are used on Medicare patients and mean we charge them for the water they drink. The charge is customarily capped at a gallon per day. You have to put it on a miscellaneous charge slip."

The secretary bought it and wrote out the charge slip. Several minutes later, having ducked out of sight and into the lunchroom, I rummaged through a cupboard for a cracker to hold me over until someone could relieve me for lunch.

"Holy moly, it's almost ten o'clock. I'm famished," a voice behind me whined. It was Chloe, whose reputation for an insatiable appetite was already legendary. She was constantly grazing.

"Didn't have any breakfast, Chloe?"

"Yeah, I had a big breakfast. Should have brought a snack, I guess. Any more crackers in that box?"

"Sure." I handed her the box of saltines, knowing there were only two crackers left. Looking in the refrigerator, I spied a casserole and remembered the lovely potluck of international cuisine we'd all enjoyed the day before. "There's some leftover casserole in this dish here. Why don't you grab some of it?"

Chloe opened the lid and placed the dish in the microwave, set the power level to reheat, grabbed a fork from the utensil drawer, gobbled up the casserole, and made it back out to her desk to man the phone in six minutes flat.

It felt good to be able to help the personnel assigned to my charge. I'd do anything for them. Almost three weeks earlier, I had confiscated a whole Chinese buffet cart from an empty conference room. The cart was loaded with all sorts of culinary delights, and I couldn't imagine letting such a gold mine go to waste.

Nurse Marie was a bit suspicious at my appearance with the cart, and, after first downing a few egg rolls and a mound of chicken-fried rice, she asked, "Ray, did you say you *bought* this for us?"

"No, Marie," I answered. "I *brought* this for you."

Having descended upon the feast, the other nurses made short work of my gift. The look Marie gave me convinced me to return the cart to the cafeteria through the back hall, just in case I'd been wrong in my assumption the conference attendees had gotten a chance to partake.

An hour and a half after Chloe finished off the casserole, I bumped into Nurse Stephanie while retrieving a chart.

"Hey, Ray! You don't happen to know what happened to my lunch, do you? It's not in the refrigerator, where I put it this morning."

"What was it?" I asked, still feeling a pang of guilt for having been caught red-handed with my fork in the last casserole she had brought in for a potluck. (I had tried to put the blame on Dr. King's desire to know what spices she'd used, but Nurse Stephanie was nobody's fool.)

"I packed some of my Italian casserole I made for yesterday's potluck and brought it back in for my lunch."

"Oh. Chloe ate it," I said without flinching.

Nurse Stephanie stormed off to find Chloe, and I got out my wallet in preparation for an anticipated act of contrition. As for writing out more miscellaneous charge slips for "no free water" patients, Chloe was reoriented correctly within a few weeks, and in time she came to forgive my little joke.

In my early days as a charge nurse, I rented a camp some thirty miles from the hospital. It was not the Hyatt Regency, but it did have two rooms—a bedroom and a bathing/living/eating/entry/kitchen (affectionately dubbed "BLEEK") room. There was electricity but no running water or heating system. It was a real steal year round for $25.00 a month.

One auspicious thing the cabin did have was a four-paned window in the bedroom, which I noticed before signing any lease. I subsequently removed one top pane of this window, installed a metal plate with a circular insert, and ran the metal pipe for a woodstove through the insert. This allowed me to lay in my bed, lean over, open the woodstove door, throw a log on the fire, and be back in REM land in a little under sixty seconds. When I went away for any extended amount of time, I gathered up anything liquid in the camp and put it in the refrigerator to keep it from freezing.

After five years of such luxurious surroundings, I left this camp. A bachelor friend of mine from nursing school, Nurse Dean, took it over and enjoyed it for the next four years. The first time I went to see him out there, I walked into my lovely BLEEK room and found Nurse Dean in the process of splitting logs right there on the floor. This was home improvement at its best.

While I was still living in the camp, the lack of shower facilities forced me to make other arrangements to support my hygiene. At least three to four times each week, I showered and washed my hair at various facilities in the area. One such place was a shower facility at the hospital where I worked. It was by the elevator just off the psych ward, and I had obtained permission to use it from the department head of that ward.

During one of my shower adventures near the psych ward, as I was shutting off the water and watching the last bit of rinse circle the drain, I heard just outside the door the unmistakable clickety-clack of high heels going back and forth. This was either a woman or a transvestite, I thought. Then someone cleared her voice from behind the closed door. It reminded me of one of my favorite poems ("Poem") by Leonard Cohen, in which a man clears his throat outside a door to a room in which another man is lying with a beautiful woman.

I wrapped my towel around me, quickly gathered my belongings, and fumbled for the doorknob. In my haste, I dropped my towel in the doorway. As I stood back up, I found myself staring down the barrels of a pair of forty-four double *D*s and had an uneasy feeling a shotgun blast was not far behind.

My six-foot frame now fully erect, I stood face to face with what I was up against. With her stout arms perched upon her hips, the double *D*s had gone into high beam. I took a quick nurse assessment of the enemy: hair tightly drawn into a knot; fire-engine red lipstick; yellow stains in her armpits; starched white uniform with a steely belt holding up the barrels; white pantyhose on legs that would have put Erik the Red to shame. It was dreadful. *Oh rats,* my inner voice screamed.

"Next?" I offered, thinking a bit of humor might help.

"Don't you know this is a locked ward? What are you doing out of it?" the voice demanded. Removing from around her neck a red lanyard holding a key to the ward, she unlocked the door.

"I work here. I'm a charge nurse---"

"Yeah, yeah, I know. And we have the hospital CEO and Jesus Christ here too."

She pushed me into the ward and slammed the door behind us. As magically as *The Wizard of Oz* went from black and white to color, I felt as if I had just entered the realm of *One Flew Over the Cuckoo's Nest.* At that moment, it dawned on me what I advised my nurses if they were ever in the presence of a psychiatrist. *Don't make eye contact,* I told them. *They can't look into your soul that way.* Taking my own bit of advice, I kept a watchful eye on those menacing B-52s, feeling sure they were capable of inflicting bodily damage.

"I've gotta hand it to you. I've seen a lot of creative ways to try and escape, but this pretty much beats 'em all."

The department head who had granted me permission was away that day, and it was only after several phone calls (and laughs on the other end)---plus a lot of checking---that I finally convinced Nurse "Ratched" I was indeed who I said I was. Not surprisingly, I never again showered in that facility or, for that matter, went anywhere near the psych floor.

Physical nakedness, along with not being heard, has a way of increasing one's sense of vulnerability in any given situation. If the foregoing experience with loss of control had not hard-wired this concept in me as a reminder of how some patients must feel, I was about to learn it all over again.

Dr. N was an orthopedic surgeon who had fallen on hard times during his life. He told me that during the Korean War he was shot in the elbow "while taking a crap in the woods." After coming back to the States, recuperating, and beginning a promising career as a pediatric surgeon, Dr. N was diagnosed with a brain tumor. As he put it to me when he hired me as his groundskeeper, "My personality is in a suction canister somewhere in California." He was a bit of an odd duck but nonetheless an excellent surgeon.

Dr. N was as meticulous about his yard as he was about tying off blood vessels. His house, recently purchased for a cool two million from the owner of one of the oldest and largest retail department stores in Bangor, was widely regarded as one of the city's wealthiest estates. My instructions were to trim the grass to two and a quarter inches, weed the three flower gardens thoroughly, and water the entire grounds for forty minutes. When I finished my first day's work there, I looked around to make sure I had pulled up every weed and trimmed every blade of grass. Then I stepped into the little shower in the groundskeeper's vacant outbuilding, disrobed, and began to wash off the grime.

Within sixty seconds of the start of my shower, a loud, obnoxious alarm pierced my ears. I knew the doctor was at work and his wife was away, and I quickly rinsed the shampoo out of my hair and peeked through the ventilation holes of the shower wall. Beyond the outbuilding, a police cruiser made its way onto the tarred driveway of the mansion, and two armed policemen got out of the car and began walking in opposite directions around the house. In nursing school, we learned that some nurses can present a calm and collected demeanor in any circumstance; others are alarmists at the very least provocation. For the first and only time in my life, I joined the ranks of the latter category and backed up in panic, hitting the opposite shower wall and causing my bar of soap to tumble loudly to the floor.

"Suspect is on this side. Request backup," I heard the closer policeman speak into his little walkie-talkie thing.

"Don't shoot!" I yelled, trying to get a hold of myself. "Hey, man, I'm just taking a shower."

"Out with your hands up!" the first policeman commanded.

I tried to pull on my underwear, but I was still wet, and they just wouldn't cooperate.

"Come out with your hands up! Now!"

I sighed and waddled to the outside of the enclosure with my hands in the air and my underwear around my knees.

"Call Dr. N. He'll verify who I am. I was just taking a shower after working in his yard."

The other policeman found his way to his partner's side and grinned from ear to ear. "Looks like you caught someone trying to make a clean getaway," he said.

Looking over the shoulders of the two policemen, I breathed a sigh of relief as I saw Dr. N parking his Mercedes behind the cruiser.

"There he is. Ask him."

"What's going on?" Dr. N asked as he reached the two patrolmen.

"Do you know this man?"

Dr. N looked me over from head to foot. "I've never seen this man before."

"Dr. N!" I exclaimed, beginning to think Dr. N had left more than his personality in that suction canister back in California. "Don't you remember? I'm your groundskeeper. You said I could take a shower in the outbuilding when I finished."

Dr. N's mouth curled up in a little upside-down *U*, and he regarded me intently for a moment, his scarred forehead tilted sideways and his eyes squinting.

"Oh, yes. I guess I do know this fellow. Didn't recognize him without his clothes. I forgot to disable the alarm for the outbuilding before I left this morning. Sorry for your trouble, fellas."

"No problem, Dr. N," the officers said.

Turning toward me, they chuckled and added, "I guess you can go. You're clean."

Chapter 8: Moving Beyond Biases

Early in my career, there was a resident by the name of Kevyn C, and it seemed he was never where he was supposed to be. Though I had yet to meet him, we often got calls looking for him. One day, I noticed that a woman with a white coat was wearing Kevyn's name tag. After that, she came in often and always seemed to be wearing his coat.

"Is Dr. C there?" Pharmacy called and asked a few weeks later.

"No," I said, "but there's a woman here who always seems to be wearing his name tag."

Pharmacy laughed. Dr. C, it turns out, was a woman with a first name I had always associated with males. I vowed never to be tripped up by assumptions again. When the phone rang just a short time afterward, I picked it up a bit more cautiously.

"ICU. Ray speaking. How can I help you?"

"Hi, Ray. This is Nurse E. How are you this fine May morning?"

I recognized the caller as our newest Director of Nursing. "Doing great," I answered. "What can I do for you?"

"As you know, today is the first day of Nurses Week. Is there a particularly deserving nurse there whom I could take to coffee with me today?"

"I'm sure that would be very much appreciated, especially since many of our staff rarely get to have much time for lunch, let alone coffee. All of our staff are deserving. Let me see who might be available."

"I'd like to go in about ten minutes."

"I'll have someone meet you at the cafeteria in ten then."

"Thank you. Ta-ta!"

Ta-ta? I shrugged it off and scanned the schedule, locating a nurse I felt had a relatively flexible load.

"Nurse Kathy, the Director of Nursing wants to take a nurse to coffee in ten minutes. Can you swing that and meet her at the cafeteria?"

"Sure can. I just finished up with my patient in Room 141."

Though she wouldn't have to pay for her coffee, Kathy felt obliged to follow the rules and to make the treat less expensive for her host by wearing her name tag. In those days, wearing a name tag was the only way to ensure a discount. Having left her name tag in her locker several rooms away, Kathy asked Nurse Theresa if she could borrow hers.

"Sure," Theresa said, handing Kathy her name tag before popping into a patient's room to answer an alarm. Kathy pinned the name tag to her coat and headed for the cafeteria.

Kathy found the Director standing patiently in front of the cafeteria and smiled pleasantly at her. "It's so nice to meet you, E," Kathy offered, extending her hand. "Thank you for treating me to coffee."

E glanced down at Kathy's name tag and in her sophisticated and always well-informed way proclaimed, "I have heard so many wonderful things about you, Theresa. I've been following your career, and I can see that you are going to do great things here at the medical center."

Being the classy woman she was, Kathy didn't let on that she was not Theresa.

A few months later, Kathy was in charge when she got a call that JACHO and Director of Nursing E wanted a tour of the ICU. Kathy made sure there were no drinks at the nursing station and reminded her staff to wipe the powdered-sugar donut crumbs off their lips and don their name tags. Before lanyards came into vogue, nurses often preferred not to pin name tags to their coats because of the possibility of being ripped out by a patient in crisis. Staff quickly picked up name tags from the desk, and Kathy pinned one to her coat before sweeping any remaining tags into a drawer below.

The Director of Nursing, a bit nervous about wanting to make a good impression on the accrediting agency and on her staff, arrived in the unit with her entourage a few minutes later.

"What's your name?" the Director whispered to Kathy.

Realizing that her lapel partially hid her name tag, Kathy adjusted her name tag so that the Director could read it.

The Director's eyes grew wide. "Better keep that covered," she said.

The inspection went off without a hitch, and JACHO left satisfied that the ICU was meeting standards for patient safety and care. In the quiet moments that followed the group's departure, Kathy unpinned her name tag and opened the drawer where the unclaimed ones had been hastily stashed.

Nurse Roger happened by at that moment. "Hey, I have something for you," he said, unpinning a name tag from his coat. He handed her a name tag with the name *Kathy* on it, and she handed him the one she'd unwittingly worn with the name *Roger* on it.

"For each life is a book, not to be read, but rather a story to be written."
~Max Luca, clergyman, writer

Though Bangor is a city of fewer than 40,000, its location has made it an ideal spot for an international airport since the late 1960s. Bangor was the first American soil soldiers returning from Afghanistan reached, and, sometimes---especially in the event of a security threat, mechanical difficulty, or medical emergency---it is the first stopover for travelers from Europe.

According to news accounts, on one such flight, a woman, whose flight had originated in Africa and had made connections in Paris with a destination of New York City, suddenly became violently ill. The flight was detained until the woman could be removed to our hospital, where she was first seen in the ER. Since there was no time to clear customs, the police closely monitored the situation. In a city that rarely sees the excitement of an unsolved mystery, the police also seemed to revel in the possibility they could be dealing with espionage.

Staff scurried to determine the cause of the woman's symptoms. The differential included diabetes, hypothyroidism, thyroid crisis, and cancer, all of which carried potentially serious risk. As was also reported by the local papers, during the course of an abdominal X-ray series, little spherical images were detected. One of these spheres appeared to have burst, spilling its contents into the woman's intestines. After further analysis, medical staff concluded the woman had swallowed about fifty little bags of cocaine, and the police who had escorted her from the airport quickly put two and two together. Narcotics and synthetic drugs have complicated the landscape with which law enforcement, as well as nurses, must deal. We've seen a patient who bled out after ripping out his own testicles and one who used a paring knife to cut out her own teeth; both were under the influence of bath salts.

Nurse Amber was the African woman's nurse in the ER and accustomed to dealing with patients from the local jail. A guard often accompanied such patients. If the inmate was violent or a prior escapee, two or more guards would accompany the patient. On this occasion, two guards resembling Andy and Barney on the Andy Griffith Show now proceeded to handcuff the woman's hands to the side rails of the stretcher. When the woman started to vomit, Amber instinctively knew she needed to be turned onto her side, and she asked the guards to remove one of the handcuffs. They felt around in their pockets for the key.

"I think the key is out in the squad car," one of them finally said.

"Well, Mutt and Jeff, she's vomiting, and I have to turn her on her side. Do you think you could get the freakin' key, or do you want to deal with the consequences?"

Nurses would never be allowed to be so careless as to lose a key, and Amber's patience had run thin. Later, she would be called into the office to face their complaint about lack of respect, but she had made her point and did succeed in getting the handcuff unlocked and her patient turned to prevent aspiration.

The woman was subsequently moved to ICU. Because the police were required to preserve a chain of evidence in the case, they maintained vigil outside this patient's room and waited patiently for the woman to stool. We had given her medications to promote evacuation, and the nurses were delighted to be able to pass the bedpans off to the police, who assumed the unpleasant task of straining the contents. Having been responsible for bedpans every day of our careers, it felt cathartic to be able to share the wealth.

When the police tried to question this African woman, she indicated she "no speak-a da English." We nurses, on the other hand, passed no judgment upon the woman, treated her like a human being, shared the universal language of a smile, and were soon able to learn that her name was Chidiebete, which in African means "God is merciful." She was the single mother of twelve children, two of whom had contracted AIDS. So thankful and trusting was her attitude toward us that she would frequently kiss our hands after speaking with us. She wept when telling us about feeling trapped into transporting the cocaine. She was paid $1,000 to do this, which for her amounted to two years of income, enough to feed her children and provide the medical care so crucial to their survival.

"Shh," we'd say. "We don't want to know because we don't want to have to testify against you."

It was wrong, sure. No question. Bringing more drugs into the community for distribution to our children is not a good thing. But the way most of us saw it, our children have a choice, and making such choices start at home. They have a chance. What chance did Chidiebete's children have without her desperate attempt? How far would *we* have gone to save *our* children? The police called her a "mule." We saw her simply as a "mother."

I've always been impressed with a nurse's ability to ignore a patient's history and provide unconditional care to anyone who comes through our doors. We once cared for a man who was shot and apprehended by police after he had shot and killed his own little child in a custody battle. When he arrived in our ICU, we treated him (as we treated Chidiebete) like he was the most important person in the world.

Moving beyond biases and leaving such baggage at the door is sometimes difficult and personal, but it is always necessary if our care is to be transformative. Again, it is crucial to burn ourselves completely, leaving no smoke to obscure our mission. A most powerful lesson in avoiding biases came when Dr. King related the story of a young woman in his church whom he had initially avoided because of a series of very extensive, colorful tattoos that he couldn't help but notice by virtue of a low-cut blouse she wore. The tattoos started at her collarbone and extended down below where her cleavage started.

"What's this all about?" the doctor asked, pointing at the tattoos and unable to contain his disgust upon seeing what he perceived at that time to be a form of self-mutilation, an adulteration of one of God's gifts.

"Ten years ago," the woman began, "four of my children were attending a birthday party for their cousin. Afterwards, I sent my oldest child to pick them up. A tactor-trailer truck struck their vehicle and killed all my children instantly. Rather than burying my heart with them, I chose to have their five sweet faces tattooed next to my heart. I will carry them with me forever."

"But one man loved the pilgrim soul in you, and loved the sorrows of your changing face."
~W.B. Yeats, poet

Nurses are trained to be very perceptive. Any subtle change in a patient's color, any misplaced word or gesture, any small detail—missed by most others---can be glaringly apparent to one so trained. Add to this the trust a focused nurse imparts to a patient, and the opportunity exists to learn a great deal.

In the spring of 1982, firemen were called to a house on a back road in Skowhegan. Mrs. Thompson was found in the partially burned dwelling, the apparent victim of a fatal gunshot wound. Mr. Thompson landed in the ICU because of burns.

I was assigned to be the primary nurse for Mr. Thompson, but I was not privy to the circumstances preceding his admission. Almost immediately upon my first encounter with him, I noticed a perfectly round burned spot on my patient's wrist. By my second day with him, we had formed a pretty good rapport with one another.

"How did you happen to burn your wrist in a perfect circle?" I asked.

I was surprised when Mr. Thompson began to tell me in great detail all that had transpired the morning he was burned. Not until later did I conclude that his regret, conscience, and trust in me had likely played a role in his spilling the beans.

"I poured gasoline into the tub to start a fire. When I lit it, the explosive force caused one of the round shower rings to land on my wrist."

"Why did you want to start a fire in the first place?"

"My wife went out the night before, and I was pretty sure she was up to no good. Anyway, I ended up putting a bullet between her eyes. She deserved it—don't you worry 'bout that.'"

I continued hanging an IV bag, trying my best not to react. Years of living with teenagers and trying to maintain their trust and confidence had taught me such a skill.

"I thought the best way to avoid prison was to burn the evidence," he continued. "Only trouble was the fire fighters happened to be at a meeting just a few blocks down the street and put the fire out too quickly to cover anything up."

Since I had been his primary nurse, I was later called as a witness for the Prosecution. Apparently, if the Defense could have proven that I had diagnosed the wrist wound as a burn, the case would have been thrown out of court, since nurses are prohibited from diagnosing.

"No," I simply answered during questioning. "I knew it was a burn. I was just curious as to how it happened, which Mr. Thompson related to me in detail."

"Heat not a furnace for your foe so hot that it do singe yourself."
~William Shakespeare, *King Henry the Eighth*

Treat everyone with the same respect and care. Whether someone is a VIP or a drug abuser, they should both be treated with respect. There are times when a nurse may be disrespectful to a patient addicted to drugs. We are not here to judge---we know nothing about their life, how it started out, and what they have been through. Comfort them and be kind.

~ Anna Montejano, RN

Nurse Colleen was a rookie when she came to work in the ICU. It was a traumatic introduction to the craft of nursing, analogous to total immersion in the deep end of a pool for someone who had never seen water.

"I'm not taking care of that SOB in 147!" she informed me one dark, rainy morning after shift change.

The passive-aggressive nonverbal of her loudly clicking, leather-soled shoes underlined Colleen's anger. I watched her stomp away from me and plop herself in a chair by one of the nursing station windows. For a moment it seemed as if there was a reflection of the windowpane upon her face, but it was tears---not rain---I was seeing.

I'd stood in Colleen's shoes before and understood her anger. Several years earlier, a man had come into our unit after sustaining a head injury in a motorcycle crash, and his care demanded a lot of our time and resources.

"Riders who don't bother with helmets should stand at the back of the line," I'd asserted.

Nurse Dean set me straight. "All patients are in need of our compassion, Ray."

Dean had taught me a lot about presencing over the years, and I sighed, knowing he was right and conceding there were still a few lessons I needed to learn.

"Who lit the fuse on Colleen's tampon?" Nurse Sherri asked.

I shrugged my shoulders, walked to the windows and sat down next to her. "He's kind of rough, huh?" I opened.

For a moment there was only the sound of the rain. "He's a drug dealer," Colleen finally said. "My sister died from a drug overdose. Why should I lift one finger to help someone like him?"

I put my head down and put my hand on her shoulder.

"It doesn't seem fair, does it?" I thought about the recent bombing at the Boston Marathon and marveled at how my fellow nurses in Boston could care for Dzhokhar Tsarnaev as professionally as if he were one of the young victims of his crime.

"May I please have a different assignment? Give me anything else, but I can't do this one," Colleen pleaded.

That morning, I took this patient myself, giving Colleen some time to pull herself together. "This won't be the last time you'll feel this way toward a patient. It's a hard pill to swallow, but you need to rise above your biases. Try to remember that this patient, after all, was once a little kid, precious in our sight. After lunch, I expect you'll be able to relieve me."

Lunch came and went, and so did Colleen. She made her point by going home "sick." What she didn't expect was that I was not going to let her off the hook and allow her emotional intelligence to plateau at the incontinence level. It didn't take long for the other staff members to notice I had taken on more than my fair share due to Colleen's inability to take this patient. I carried not only my charge duties but also half of her responsibilities. Peer pressure is a powerful thing.

The next morning, Colleen breezed past me without saying a word. *Oh, the silent treatment,* I thought to myself, noting she had just left 147 with a urine sample. *At least she's going to give it a try.*

I kept a close eye on Room 147 that day and the days following. Though this was a challenge I wanted Colleen to meet, I could not allow patient care to suffer as a consequence. Nothing could have prepared me for the transformation about to take place.

"Nurse, could I have my pain meds? It's past time and hurts like hell."

"That's the idea, Shithead," she mumbled under her breath.

"What?"

"Let me adjust your bed," she said.

"Pain meds?" Gerald asked again, looking her squarely in the eyes.

"Oh, yes, I'll be right back with them."

Almost ten minutes later, Colleen returned with his pain medications. Gerald was curled up in a ball in the middle of his bed. I walked in and noticed his discomfort.

"How're things going?" I asked.

Before Colleen could answer, Gerald looked up and smiled.

"Great," he replied. "My nurse is an angel on Earth."

I winked at Colleen, whose hands were still suspended over the IV pump. She smiled nervously and continued to administer the meds.

"Jerk," she said under her breath, as I walked out the door.

"What?" Gerald said.

"Work," she said. "It's busy today. Sorry it took a while to get your meds."

"No problem. I get why you don't like me. Hell, you'd think I was used to it by now. But you don't even know me, and you hate me. Heck, I hate me . . . Thanks for getting my meds."

Gerald was thirty-something but looked like sixty. He turned his graying head toward the window and stared at the river scene outside. Colleen's hatred subsided long enough to let in a little pity.

"Thanks for rising to the occasion," I said to Colleen later that day. "Sometimes we just have to bite the bullet and realize we need to treat everyone with the same respect and kindness. Otherwise, it will destroy us."

Colleen smiled at me and went on with her duties. It was obvious she hadn't completely bought this, but it was a start.

Later that week we got another admission. Another person who sold illegal drugs. The only difference upon first glance at his chart was that this person, a nationally renowned business executive, was considered a VIP. Later a second difference would emerge: this guy was a royal pain in the butt. One can measure the caring capability of a hospital by the policies it sets forth regarding the treatment of VIPs; such treatment should be no different, no more and no less, than the treatment afforded any other patient who comes through its doors.

Colleen almost didn't notice the little figure at the back of Gerald's room when she went in to pick up his tray after lunch. The young girl was perched upon the high-backed, green leather chair common to all the rooms, and she looked like a doll.

"Hi," the young girl said. "Are you helpin' to make my papa better?"

"Of course," Colleen said. "What's your name?"

"Kristin," she said. "When can he come home? Me 'n my brother miss him."

"I don't know---where's your mom?"

"She went to live with Jesus after Papa got laid off. Papa said if I'm good, I'll get to see her again."

A lump formed in Colleen's throat. "How did you get here?"

"A nice man from the shelter brought me. He's waitin' in the waitin' room for me. I promised I wouldn't be too long. How come Papa doesn't have lobster like the man across the hall? I saw them bring it into him, and he didn't even say 'thank you.' Papa told me sayin' 'thank you' was proper."

Colleen glanced over at Gerald, whose moist eyes were fixed on his little girl. She checked the monitors, adjusted Gerald's pillow, glanced in the mirror, and turned back to the little girl.

"Some people just can't see past themselves enough to appreciate what they have," she answered.

That night Gerald enjoyed a lobster dinner with all the trimmings that usually accompany a Down East feast. Colleen had made the arrangements and also arranged for Kristin and her brother to come for another visit. Gerald was very grateful.

"I'm tryin' real hard," he said to her the next day. "Them kids is all I got, but I got to do right by them. You showed me there's still kindness in the world. I just hafta hang in there till I can find work again. Thanks for believing in me."

Colleen had been swept into an undertow of understanding and had arrived in a calm sea of acceptance. Gone were the anger, the spite, and the revenge. *We all have our crosses to bear*, she thought to herself. *My sister had hers; Gerald has his; I have mine. Some of us just need more help than others to carry the load.*

"Oh, one more thing," Gerald added. "I happened to see on my chart where you checked off 'SOB' every hour for a few days last week . . ."

"It stands for 'shortness of breath,'" she offered quickly and smiled. "Nothing more."

"When you change the way you look at things, the things
you look at change."
~Dr. Wayne W. Dyer, author, motivational speaker

Critical care nurses may also develop biases about the relatively minor injuries of people outside the intense, life-and-death struggles of the intensive care unit. Similarly, people who discover that someone is a nurse or caregiver may unfairly decide that the health professional is capable of handling *any* health issue. It is important to recognize and keep the former in perspective and to set the record straight in situations that may be beyond one's capability to adequately manage in the latter. Often have I heard administration's assertion, especially in recent years when nurses were in high demand and short supply, that "a nurse is a nurse is a nurse," when in fact, each area of nursing requires a different, specialized skill set.

I sat cross-legged at the end of the examining table, my hands neatly folded over my lap. I was naked, except for my johnny tied in the back.

Dr. C, her back to me, shuffled some papers while preparing for the exam. Karen and I always made our appointments with her on the same day. "It looks like your last colonoscopy was three years ago, and because the last one looked normal, we won't have to reschedule for another seven years."

"Good," I said. "The preparation for the test is brutal. I wish they'd change it." I chuckled to myself as I thought about my history of noncompliance in preparing for colonoscopies . . .

. . . Though I always followed my patients' prescriptions to the letter, when it came to myself, I would often self-dose. When Karen tried to help me with my preparations, I told her I never took more than half of what was prescribed in a colon prep, rationalizing that I wanted to be snug in my bed, not filling a toilet bowl all night. The "end" result, I claimed, would be the same either way. I would also frequently self-refer my aftercare, a practice that probably had a lot to do with my getting fired by my first primary care physician. Upon arriving at one of my colonoscopies, a nurse who knew me well and whose charge nurse I had been five years earlier welcomed me with, "Ray, when you're in here, I'm the boss . . ."

. . . Dr. C turned around, and upon seeing me, broke into laughter. "You don't have your glasses on," she observed. "Karen just told me you make sure *she* wears *her* glasses at all times."

"Yes, because I might need to borrow hers sometime."

Dr. C chuckled, and I thought about the other habits I'd instilled in Karen since our marriage, habits she knew were extensions of my need to be prepared as a relief charge nurse in the intensive care unit for so many years. Likewise, she had learned early on not to expect a whole lot of sympathy from me as long as she was breathing and her heart was pumping.

"If you're dying, I can help you," I would often tell her. "Otherwise, I'm afraid you're on your own."

I wasn't the only critical care nurse with that mindset, and I hoped in every other way I was the compassionate and loving spouse she deserved. I thought about Nurse Carol, one of the first ICU nurses to work in our ICU and one of the first of our nurses to trade her white shoes for work boots as a flight nurse. At her retirement party we'd recently attended, it was clearly evident from the friends, family members, and fellow nurses who honored her with speeches that, like many critical care nurses, being less than sympathetic about minor injuries was her way of triaging the situation and getting on with the important stuff.

While Dr. C was engaged in my examination, the words Carol's nine-year-old grandson spoke that evening came back to me . . .

. . . "I learned many things from my nanny," he began. "She taught me songs and how to paddle a canoe . . . and I learned some neat swear words from her." The audience laughed at this, but Karen recognized that like the grandson, I also always tell it like it is, cutting right to the chase and sparing no observation. People often remark that I say what others are only thinking but dare not say. This boy had learned early on to follow his grandmother's ways.

When Carol's son Jamey next stood to speak, we strained to listen, hoping to hear more words of validation.

"When my sister Jennifer was in middle school," Carol's son began, "we took a trip to Aroostook County to celebrate Mother's Day with Mom's mom. Before we all went out to lunch, my great uncle thought it would be fun to put Jennifer on a small dirt bike and teach her how to ride it. When the throttle stuck and the bike crashed, she got thrown over the handlebars and hurt her arm. Mom looked it over, determined there was no deformity and no immediate swelling, gave her an ice bag, and---reminding her that we were going to lunch with Nana--- admonished her not to cry.

"Back in Bangor the next day, Jennifer massaged her arm in private. She confided in me that her arm hurt like hell, but she didn't want to make the painful decision to tell Mom she might have to see a doctor. Mom never liked us to cry over little bumps and bruises, and we knew she'd be mad if she saw Jennifer favoring the arm. And just in case Jennifer had any visions of getting unjustified sympathy, Mom reminded Jennifer that 'she was moving her arm, wasn't she?'

"Mom eventually noticed the extent of my sister's discomfort when Jennifer jumped onto the sideboard in an effort to reach for a glass from the cupboard. We shuffled off to the ER, where she was diagnosed with a greenstick fracture of her forearm.

"While Jennifer's arm was back to new after eight weeks in a cast, Mom never did get to live down the 'awful treatment the critical care nurse had given her daughter.' But Mom has seen a lot in her time as a nurse. When she first started, she cared for a child who had been hurt in a bike crash with a car. He was unconscious and later passed away. A sore arm on someone who was walking around just didn't seem like that big a deal to her. On the other hand, that same morning her patient died, she came home and put all our bikes away until she was sure that wasn't going to happen to us."

. . . I thought about Nurse Amy and the day a child came into our unit unresponsive after strangling on window blind cords. Amy was so concerned for the safety of her own children that she called her husband and gave him one hour to cut all the cords from their blinds.

Dr. C asked me to breathe deeply, then to exhale, as the cool cup of a stethoscope lightly touched my back. I thought about the basic tools a nurse might use to assess patients and how I often carried such tools in my car in the event I might have to help someone unexpectedly. I thought about how terribly unprepared and useless I had felt, even with such tools, because I lacked the skill set for assessing one of my friends one summer several years back. Even with all the successes I'd enjoyed with patients over the years, it was this failure that stood out and haunted me . . .

. . . In the summer of 2004, a former colleague asked if I could accompany him in a move back to Maine from Seattle. I'd made several such trips with patients and agreed to do this one. Little did I know how painfully unprepared I would be for this particular journey.

William and Hanna had lived in a nearby town for seven years, and they seemed like ordinary folk. Their children attended school with mine and often came over for a game of basketball or a jump on the trampoline. I'd sometimes run into them at PTA meetings and at church. It was with shock, then, that I read William had been charged with embezzlement at our medical office where he'd been employed as an accounts receivable clerk. Shortly afterwards, William and Hanna

265

vacated their home, and we got word they'd moved out west near her parents in an attempt to evade the charges. I thought the crime and their actions odd but was not aware then that William had an underlying, contributing problem.

A year later, we received a phone call from Hanna telling us she'd convinced William to come back and face charges. If I could help him with a large U-Haul of belongings, as well as a car in tow, then Hanna and the kids would fly back. I agreed to help my friends, and they arranged a one-way flight for me through Chicago to Seattle. Hanna met me in the driveway when my taxi dropped me off.

"William's packed and unpacked the U-Haul a couple of times since yesterday. Thanks for coming."

I chalked up William's uncertainty about leaving to his fear of what lay ahead in Maine. It was understandable. Later, at Hanna's parents' home, however, I got the full story.

"My son-in-law graduated top of his class from Harvard in economics," Hanna's father said during a quiet moment alone with me. "Very smart man. Terrible what can happen to people, isn't it?"

"What do you mean?" I asked.

"Didn't they tell you? He's got OCD. And he's bipolar. On Trazodone every day. Otherwise, well, you know." And he made circular motions with his fingers in front of his ear.

I had dealt with patients with obsessive compulsive disorder (OCD) a few times and knew I might have my work cut out for me. If Hanna had been upfront with me earlier, I could've been a whole lot better prepared than I was.

We planned a very early departure the next morning, hoping to get a jump on the four thousand miles ahead of us. But William said he needed more time to think about whether or not he was making the right decision in moving back. By 10:00 am, I was drumming my fingers on the kitchen table, while William and Hanna were discussing things in the bedroom. Finally, Hanna's younger daughter spoke up.

"Daddy, please leave," she said.

William came out into the kitchen, put on his baseball cap, and said we'd better get going. I didn't wait around until he changed his mind but hopped into the passenger side of the large U-Haul, behind which was hitched his '87 Chevy. He drove down Interstate 90 at a hesitant forty to forty-five miles per hour to the Washington state border, at which point clouds of doubt again surfaced and we discussed his desire to turn back. This conversation was interrupted by frequent stops—stops to make phone calls to Hanna, stops to use a bathroom, and stops to fuel the truck (made the more frequent because he would put in only half a tank of gas at each stop). Seven hours and only 290 miles after leaving Seattle, William wanted to put up for the night. I talked him into letting me drive 167 more miles to Missoula, Montana before calling it a night.

Just after nine o'clock, I climbed into my motel bed and shut my eyes, knowing the next day would likely hold more of the same challenges. It wasn't long before I felt a light thump on my bed and then a swish of fur against my head. William had failed to tell me we were transporting a cat in the back of the truck, and he had brought it into the motel room.

"William," I said softly.

Loud snoring was the only response. I brushed the cat off the bed and turned back to my pillow, only to sense the same thump-swish, again requiring me to brush the creature off the bed. Our interactions were repeated several times before I lost my patience and woke up William.

"The cat has to go. Lock it in the bathroom or in the truck or something, but it has to go."

He closed it in the bathroom, where it meowed the entire night. Cats had never been high on my list of favorites, and by morning they were several notches lower.

The next morning, William insisted on having breakfast at a local diner, and he spent close to three hours sipping his coffee, while I finished off an English muffin topped with crunchy peanut butter and orange marmalade.

"We have to get on the road," I insisted, nervously watching the clock. He sighed, put on his cap, and slid into the driver's seat. As we headed out of Missoula, I noticed him turn west on I-90 toward Seattle.

"Oh, you're going the wrong way," I said, giving him the benefit of the doubt he'd made a mistake. "You're going west now, and you want to go east."

He didn't say a word but stared straight ahead, apparently bent on returning. My thoughts retreated to my high school Latin class, where I learned to conjugate the Latin verb *delirare*, which means "to go off track." In college I learned that *delirare* was the origin of the English word *delirious*, and now I was appreciating that little tidbit of trivia more than ever before.

"You can go back to Seattle if you want to, but I'm not going. You can let me off here, and I'll get a ride home." I thought this little tactic might nudge William into compliance, but he continued driving, saying nothing for almost an hour.

Finally, he turned the truck eastward. By this time, I was getting a sense William was delaying his trip to Maine. It was clear I needed to take a different tack if we were to ever make it back home. It was touch-and-go as we watched Butte, Billings, and Sioux Falls retreat one by one in our rearview mirrors. When we reached Chicago, William knew this was the halfway point, and he likely felt it represented the point of no return. His insecurities intensified, and he made more frequent stops to call Hanna, always indicating he needed more time to think about things.

As William kept insisting upon driving, I made a large sign to keep things light and to encourage him. On it in large letters I wrote "Maine," and it made him laugh. As we passed the city limits of Cleveland, I sensed he wanted to stop, and I held up my sign. He smiled. Ten minutes later, we were stopped at a phone booth. After several hours of William trying to reach Hanna, I called my wife from another booth.

"Hanna and the kids flew out early," my wife said. "She couldn't take the phone calls anymore."

Great, I thought to myself, for the first time understanding that William probably feared Hanna would leave him. I walked back to the other phone booth and rapped on the door.

"Hey, man, Hanna's already in Maine! She wanted to surprise you, so don't tell her I gave it away. She's staying at my house."

As he stood there staring at me, I began to fear for my life. If I'd been trained in psychiatric medicine, I would've known that the mentally ill are victims of violent crime more often than perpetrators of it. But lacking this understanding, I succumbed to the irrational fear that accompanies ignorance. This man looked as if he would shortly lose more than the toy he'd joked about missing from his Happy Meal. I thought he needed some direction.

"William, you have three choices. You can continue on to Maine with me; you can go back to Seattle; or you can go to a clinic. I'm continuing on—I won't go to Seattle with you—so if you decide later you want to go back to Maine with me, call your wife to find out where I'm at."

I thrust out my thumb to begin hitchhiking to a motel we'd seen two exits back. William left the phone booth and stood next to me.

"Get away from me. I can't get a ride with you standing here."

He noticed my uneasiness and suggested a Trazodone. Then he got into the U-Haul and started down the interstate ramp, only to make a quick U-turn and circle back to where I was standing. He circled back to me repeatedly until I was able to get a ride with a gentleman who looked harmless. In fact, he turned out to be a pizza deliveryman from my hometown in Maine, and he kindly drove me to a Motel 6.

Later that night, as I lay my head against my pillow and looked forward to some peace and quiet, William knocked on my door. He had found me at the motel after calling my wife. I had been feeling very inadequate as a nurse, unable to handle this situation, and his return to me made me feel somewhat like the welcoming father upon his prodigal son's return. At the same time, I felt like God's faithful, yet tortured, servant Job, who, having endured the destruction of his children and worldly possessions, as well as having been covered from head to toe in loathsome sores, retired to sit in the ashes, scraping his sores with a piece of broken pottery, and cursing the day he was born.

The next day, his pleas to turn back with him became so frequent during our drive that I penned the word "NO" on the flip side of my "Maine" sign and held it up whenever William hesitated. My head hurt so badly from the constant badgering that I began popping Tylenol like candy.

"Would you go back to Seattle with me?"

I held up my sign: "NO."

Ten minutes later, he repeated his question for the twentieth time that hour.

"F*** you, William!"

I had reached the limit of my humanity, or perhaps I had only reverted to my most human state. At any rate, I knew my cardboard sign was no longer helping either of us stay grounded. I gave William three new choices: call ahead for hotel reservations in a town 300 miles away; let me drive; or go to the town up ahead. Otherwise, I would be hitchhiking back by myself, and he could do whatever he wanted. William decided he would be brave and try to go back to Seattle on his own. He dropped me off at the next motel and turned the U-Haul around. I watched the dust fly up around his truck as he headed west, shook my head with disbelief at how I was spending my summer vacation, and went inside to book a room for the night. It was already 7:00 pm, and I dialed my wife to fill her in on what was happening.

"William's on the other line," she said after many rings. "He said he made you mad."

"What's the number he's calling from?"

I recognized the phone number as originating from the same phone booth where we'd spent several hours the day before.

"Ask him if he would get a room for the night and consider meeting me at McDonald's in Bay Village tomorrow morning at 7:00."

William was sitting at a table when I arrived at McDonald's at the appointed time. One thing I've noticed about accountants is they're always on time.

"Ray, I need to have you travel with me. It's too scary by myself."

"Okay," I said, "But you're gonna have to get a room by yourself. Otherwise, there'll be two of us on Trazodone."

William insisted on driving the first leg. He seemed to hug the line separating the lanes, forcing passing traffic onto the shoulder, and his inattention forced me to demand my spot back behind the wheel. That night we managed to reach Boston, where I agreed to share the same room with him, as long as he agreed to do something different with the cat. Later, when I was sure he was asleep, I sneaked out of the room and walked down the hall to the lobby, where I dialed the telephone number for a local hospital and asked to speak to the charge nurse on the psych ward. He helped me to understand OCD and bipolar disorder better, but he also told me I wasn't responsible for William's welfare. More than halfway home, I now felt a little better prepared to see it through.

The following morning, William again insisted on driving. He knew he would be arriving in Maine that evening, and this was perhaps his last attempt at some control. Reluctantly, I slid onto the passenger side seat. We sat together in the parking lot from 7:30 am until 10:30 am, William sipping a coffee and studying the map. He seemed to be staring a hole right through the atlas, and something the charge nurse had said suddenly made sense. Inattention and inability to focus may have been indications that William was not taking his medication, and I asked him if he'd swallowed the Trazodone I'd been giving him.

"I've been cheeking it for the last four or five days," he admitted victoriously.

Everything started to make sense: the anxiety about the trip, the packing and unpacking, the inability to make decisions, going the wrong way, the constant pestering about turning around, the erratic driving and loss of focus. When William went into the motel's restroom, I went into the police barracks, which happened to be right across the street, told them I feared for my life, and was told they could not help me unless we were involved in a crash. I also contacted the local medical clinic, which directed me to a mental health clinic. Two people from the Mobile Crisis Unit met us in the parking lot and evaluated William. They encouraged him to take his Trazodone and then gave him choices similar to what I had offered the day before: Ray could drive both of them; William could drive himself, in which case they would help me get a motel and fly me back the rest of the way; or William could go to a hospital. After three hours of slow, painful, unmedicated thinking, William made the decision to let me drive.

As we crossed the bridge from Portsmouth, New Hampshire into Maine, William became more agitated. Though we were less than four hours from home, I wanted desperately to get some Trazodone into William.

"How 'bout a Moxie?" I asked. We'd stopped briefly at a greasy spoon, and I figured he'd be thirsty.

"Okay."

When I brought our drinks back to the truck, he'd switched to the driver's seat, but I felt as if I were one up on him. I'd already opened the bottles and added a crushed tablet of his medication to one of the otherwise identical drinks. He looked at me suspiciously, then thanked me and took a sip.

"You didn't add something to this, did you?" he asked.

"What are you talking about?" I responded, not wanting to lie.

He smiled, then took my bottle from the dash cup holder, did a little switching extravaganza with the bottles, and placed them both back in the holders. I didn't know for sure which drink contained the medication, so I focused on our being only about four hours from our destination. Still, every time I took a sip, I wondered.

When we finally turned onto the road where I lived, I thought I would burst with the anticipation that my nightmare was almost over and that I could go back to being a nurse in ICU, not the psych ward. There was a snowmobile clubhouse less than half a mile from my home, and William steered the truck into the parking lot there and stopped.

So close.

"Can we turn back?" he asked.

In disbelief, all I could do was to hold up my sign: "NO."

William reached into his pocket. *Please, God, don't let us die here*, I prayed under my breath, my hand on the door handle. He pulled out his battery-operated shaver and proceeded to shave his face.

"I've got to look presentable for my family," he said. William was a handsome man and usually presented himself well. He pulled out a comb and ran it through his head of thick blond hair. "Just one last thing," he said, reaching into his other pocket.

I clenched my teeth, thinking this might be it, but he pulled out a Trazodone and popped it into his mouth with what was left of the Mt. Dew. "Give me thirty minutes to reach equilibrium, okay?"

William's family was impressed with my getting him to them in such good physical shape. I, on the other hand, arrived mired in uncertainty. Haggard from sleeping with one eye open, I had gone from being confident at the start of the trip---having, after all, been the proud first recipient of the medical center's Nurse of the Year Award---to being disillusioned about my skills as a caregiver. When I opened my journal that evening and described how I'd spent my summer vacation, I was relieved to end the entry with, "Tomorrow I will be returning to the ICU, where for a moment . . . I will feel so certain."

It was the last time I agreed to help transport a psych patient, but it also reminded me about the many disciplines within the field of nursing. One is lucky to be able to become proficient in a couple of them in a lifetime and foolish to believe one could master them all. Next time such a situation presented itself, I was quick to suggest someone trained in the discipline of psychiatric caregiving . . .

. . . I dressed and bid farewell to Dr. C until my next checkup. I felt confident Dr. C had the training to recognize anything amiss about my health, and I was glad I'd entrusted my care to her rather than to a pediatrician.

"What lies behind us and what lies before us are tiny matters compared to what lies within us."
~Ralph Waldo Emerson, philosopher

Chapter 9: The Psych Patient

Nursing care comes in many forms. Sometimes it is the ability to make someone feel physically comfortable by various means. Other times it is the ability to improve the body's ability to achieve or maintain health. But often it is an uncanny yet well-honed knack to see beyond the obvious and address, in some way, the deeper needs of the human soul.

~Donna Wilk Cardillo[15]

According to Albert Einstein, "There are only two ways to live your life. One is as though nothing is a miracle. The other is as though everything is a miracle." I have never seen a miracle. That doesn't mean they don't happen. We've all heard stories about tumors spontaneously disappearing. Medicine has come a long way since the days of Hippocrates, but it is still far from being an exact science. How many times have you or a loved one gone to a doctor, only to be told you have a "virus"? That's sometimes a physician's way of circumnavigating uncertainty about what is wrong with you. You are told that it will clear up in about a week or two and you must simply wait for it to pass. Nine times out of ten it does.

In the same way some of our physical ailments seem to defy explanation by modern medicine, there exist in history examples of phenomena that have, after exhaustive investigation, no satisfactory explanations. Documented accounts of individuals disappearing seemingly into thin air, sometimes in front of others, abound.

Though hardened cynics can almost always come up with an explanation for such phenomena, it is much more difficult to explain *multiple* disappearances. In November of 1930, a fur trapper made his way on snowshoe to a village of more than two thousand Eskimos on the shores of Lake Anjikuni in northern Canada. When he arrived, all he found were the charred remains of a stew on a fireplace of cinders. The villagers were gone. The ensuing investigation found no footprints. Though all of the Eskimos' sled dogs had died of starvation, a good supply of food and provisions was found undisturbed in the huts. The dogs were found buried under twelve-foot snowdrifts. Even more puzzling was that the Eskimos' ancestral graves had all been emptied. Fifteen years later, a train carrying hundreds of passengers from Guandun, China disappeared without trace halfway to its destination of Shanghai.[16]

Man has characteristically attempted to assuage his discomfort with loose ends through explanations. While our ancestors may have explained away these events with mythical creatures like werewolves or fairies, the age of modern science has ushered in more sophisticated terms, such as momentary black holes, alien abduction, tears in the fabric of reality, teleportation, spontaneous combustion, and fourth dimensions. *Reality shifts*, the sudden manifestations of objects appearing, disappearing, transforming, and transporting, supposedly happen all of the time around us unnoticed. It's only when such a shift makes something noticeable (like a person or a train) disappear that we become aware of it. Many proponents of such theories note the veil separating realities appears thinnest at night. A new wave of thought in physics called *string theory* advances the idea of an infinite number of parallel universes which share space with our own dimension. ". . . In an infinite universe," writes author Dean Koontz, "anything that could be imagined might somewhere exist."[17] What force or forces prevent us from slipping into one of these other universes, dimensions, or realities?

Somewhere between fairies and parallel universes psychiatry was born. It pretends to be an evidence-based arm of medicine, but its tendency is to ignore the mosaic totality of individuals, reducing them to mere chemical pools. It rejects the idea of any consciousness existing outside the physical body, including a spirit or soul, as well as the existence of God or spiritual agents, psychic ability, aliens, the power of meditative exercises, life after death, near-death and out-of-body experiences, evil forces, reincarnation, and other dimensions and realities. Not appreciating the whole person and his or her culture strikes some as narrow-minded disservice that can lead to greater confusion and distress for a patient.

It is within this context that the mentally ill have come to reside. As a nurse, I am saddened by the inadequacy of treatments currently available for those who have been labeled as such. As research continues to disprove the efficacy of drugs---which further diminishes the idea of chemical imbalances in *all* these individuals---continuing to serve all patients with kindness and humility is vital. I share the previous story and relate the following encounters not to poke fun at the patients but to challenge others that these unfortunates are poorly underserved and deserve more open-minded attention.

Donna, a certified nursing assistant, worked in a group home. One of the residents, Orson, was a night owl. For thirty-seven years he had worked the graveyard shift at the local paper mill in Bucksport, checking for imperfections in each giant roll of paper produced. When he retired, Orson continued to sleep during the day and to prowl by night.

To keep an eye on Orson, Donna decided it would be a good idea one night to bring him to the receptionist's desk and let him watch the group home employees work and interact with each other. On the first night with them, he took a box of tissues from one of the countertops and asked if he could have it. Donna was confident Orson couldn't do much harm with a box of tissues, and she acquiesced.

"Of course. You're not catching a cold, are you?"

Orson smiled up at her and sat back down without answering. Donna went off to check on another resident.

Upon her return several minutes later, Donna noticed little white pieces of tissue paper littering the floor around where Orson sat. She walked by and turned around to watch Orson as he proceeded to take another tissue out of the box, tear it up into little pieces, and toss each piece away as if dealing out a deck of cards. Though she didn't understand what he was trying to do, she felt it was harmless and kept him occupied. At the end of her shift, Orson retired to bed and Donna swept the floor. Donna and her coworkers became accustomed to the routine, which continued for the next five nights.

Then, on one especially quiet night, the workers decided they would try to understand Orson's actions. They sat with him talking, while they systematically tore up tissues and "dealt" them out to the spaces in front of them. Orson looked at them incredulously.

"Aren't you dealing out cards?" Donna asked sincerely.

"No, Stupid," he answered. "I'm feeding the pigeons."

Because Ralph was psychotic, he presented a real challenge to all of us. We needed to treat his physical problems while keeping an eye on his mental well-being, something with which many of us had little experience. Newly oriented Nurse Julie asked me for a consult about why Ralph was having hallucinations. According to the patient's chart, Ralph had not slept since he'd been in the ICU.

Returning his chart to our lazy-Susan chart holder, I said, "Ralph's lack of rapid-eye-movement sleep and consequent lack of dreams are probably being compensated for during the daytime and being expressed as hallucinations. He hasn't slept in three nights."

A light bulb seemed to go on, and Nurse Julie, always concerned with addressing her patient's needs, gave Ralph a sympathetic look. "Are you tired?" she asked him.

As part of his hallucinations, Ralph often reported seeing spiders and scorpions in his room. Various caregivers thought they were reassuring him by arguing that the creatures were not there. By the late evening of his fourth day with us, he was still not able to sleep.

When Nurse Katy, our resident comedienne, came on duty and happened to walk by his door later that night, Ralph asked, "Nurse, do you see those spiders by the door?"

"Oh, yeah. I see them," she simply said. She entered his room and touched his arm. "Everything's fine, though. It's okay if you want to sleep."

With this simple acknowledgement of Ralph's thoughts and validation of Ralph's experience, Katy was able to calm the patient and redirect his attention, which allowed him to fall asleep. The following day, Ralph did not experience hallucinations.

When Ralph was well enough to be transferred to a psychiatric unit across town, he was placed in the care of Nurse Linda, who had recently transferred from working in the ICU. During a recreational hour one afternoon, Nurse Linda set up a game of Monopoly and invited Ralph to play.

When his game piece landed on Park Place, Nurse Linda held out her hand in anticipation of the bank's receiving payment to buy the property. "Aren't you going to buy Park Place?" she asked several minutes later, sensing no indication from Ralph that he intended to do so.

"No," he said.

Not believing her ears, Nurse Linda repeated, "You're not going to buy Park Place? Are you nuts?"

"Yes," Ralph said, without batting an eyelash.

This was one of Nurse Linda's earliest reminders that psych patients do not always present with *anosognosia*, the inability or refusal to recognize one's clinical condition.

"The greatest battles of life are fought out daily in the silent chambers of our own souls."
~David O. McKay, religious leader, educator

I watched him for several minutes before entering the room where he sat looking out the window. Every now and then he would laugh to himself and say something aloud; in the next breath he was wringing his hands in despair, his face scrunched up like a wrung wet washcloth. It seemed as if a war were being waged within his mind, and it seemed as if he should surely be torn to pieces by it. He could have been the poster child of the walking wounded from any war that ever raged.

"Hello," I said. "My name is Ray, and I'll be your nurse for the next few days. I'll do my best to help you out any way I can." (This is a phrase I had borrowed from Nurse Chris and used most of my career to communicate commitment to patients.)

"Ha!" he said, turning around to shake my hand. "Good luck with that! I'm crazy, you know."

"You have post-traumatic stress disorder---PTSD. There is a difference. I understand you've been through some heavy-duty stuff. Once we get your alcohol problem under control---"

"Were you ever in Nam?"

"No, but---"

"What could you possibly understand about an 'alcohol problem'?"

I sat down beside him, remembering my last semester in psychology class and my instructor's observation that victims of PTSD benefit from those who listen to them without passing judgment.

"I'm willing to listen. What happened in Nam?"

"What *didn't* happen? Hell, I never went any farther than the local Burger King in my hometown. All of a sudden, here I was in a friggin' jungle, tromping through swamp up to my chin and duckin' bullets all around my head." He started to sob, then looked back at me with steeled determination. "We was passin' around Demerol and pot like it was candy." He held out his hand to me and then withdrew it.

Glancing at the chart on my lap, I confirmed that *depression,* described by Sigmund Freud as "anger turned inward," was also listed as part of this unfortunate man's history. I waited patiently, until at last he continued.

"We was so full of the stuff that some of the men who got shot never knew they'd been hit. Rick, he just laid in my arms and smiled the whole time he was dyin'."

"That's rough. How'd you get it past the commander?"

"Well, see there. You don't know squat. The commander was the enemy. We got rid of probably a half dozen of *them*."

"They just couldn't take it, huh?"

"More like we couldn't take *them*. We shot most of the bastards. Funny, ain't it? They taught us to kill, and we took it to the next level. We killed women and babies and defenseless men and children . . . We killed those SOBs too. No one should force another human bein' to do those horrible things. We just couldn't take it no more." He bent over, put his head in his hands, and shook uncontrollably.

Shocked by this, I asked as gently as I could, "He was someone's son or someone's father or brother. Didn't that bother you?"

After several minutes, he continued. "Sure—at first. But it got easier—especially with the drugs. It's part of the brainwashin', you know? 'Detachment,' they call it. Which is worse: killin' babies or killin' men who order you to keep killin' babies? Doesn't the idea of killin' innocent children bother *you*? And understand—it was only the mean and rough leaders, the ones we didn't like, the ones who made us do the shit that still lives in my head—those were the ones we took out. It was easiest if we got hold of enemy weapons. Then we could make it look like they was killed by enemy fire. Sometimes we had no choice but to take 'em down when we got the chance with our own ammo. 'Friendly fire' is what they called it. Now *that's* a good one. '*Friendly* fire.'"

It wasn't the first time I'd heard about the deliberate killing of an unpopular senior officer, which is called *fragging* (since it is often accomplished with a fragmentation grenade). The almost nine hundred documented cases between 1969 and 1972 were thought to be fallout from the unpopularity of the Vietnam War and the breakdown of discipline in the armed forces.[18]

My head reeling with all I had just heard, I sat with this man for close to thirty minutes while he simply cried. Finally, looking back up at me, he opened a book that lay on his nightstand, removed a flask of

282

liquor hidden in a hollowed-out space among the pages, and handed it to me. "I want to come home," he said simply. "I want to come home."

"If you bury your feelings, you bury them alive."
~Father Powell, S.J.

Chapter 10: Final Thoughts: Psychiatrists

In dealing with those who are undergoing great suffering, if you feel "burnout" setting in, if you feel demoralized and exhausted, it is best, for the sake of everyone, to withdraw and restore yourself. The point is to have a long-term perspective.

~Tenzin Gyatso, 14th Dalai Lama

I f you hang in there long enough with nursing as a profession, you will grow to love it. You'll learn to love every wrinkle, every gray hair, every bent frame of those for whom you care. And you'll feel certain nothing else on Earth could come close to comparing with the rewards of being invited by your patient into their deepest, darkest night and emerging with the feeling you have been an integral part of a healing, transformational dawn. But, like a pressure cooker that needs to vent steam or risk blowing up, you'll also need an outlet for all the pain you will help absorb, all the heartache you will share in, all the burdens you will help lighten.

I've heard some nurses say, "The only way I can be available for *all* my patients is to do so with a guarded heart, to simultaneously protect myself. If I enter into Mr. Jones' suffering and experience the depth of a pain full of despair in the wake of certain, imminent death, how can I then possibly help Mrs. Smith find hope she can recover from her stroke?" This is the "smoky fire" Suzuki warns us about; we need to burn ourselves completely if we are to be truly accessible. We cannot hide behind our white uniform or collar or the title on our name tag that says we are a staff nurse or a charge nurse, whose duties include A, B and C, but not D. What good is being proficient in the procedures and techniques of our profession, if we fail to heal? Serving both patients fully is absolutely possible, but one must have the resolve not to run in the face of being unable to cure or fix, the courage to rise above the basic level of job or career to a higher calling, and the stamina to be there in a state that shows your patients you are as vulnerable and human as they are. I would challenge these nurses to overcome their fears and protect themselves by seeking out and using available support systems instead of escape.

One support system readily available to all but the most isolated caregiver is our network of coworkers, who can provide a sounding board for our concerns and feelings. When Colleen confided in me about her sister's death through drug abuse and her reluctance to care for a patient who was a drug dealer, she was unloading her concerns on someone who could help her cope with the situation. Such unburdening, while the other holds in confidence things revealed, is important in extending one's internal resources.

Next, try to avoid negativity. Surround yourself with positive thinkers and positive thinking. In your circle of associates include mentors, people who exhibit characteristics you admire and want to emulate. You also need at your head table not only people who believe in you and your vision when even you have lost hope, but also those supporters who would challenge that you might have strayed from your vision and who would help get you back on track. Unless you are also a skilled politician, you also need people who can foresee trouble *before* it happens and who are there to warn you about treading carefully. Lastly, you need partners who are committed to working with you and who will not undermine your efforts.

Taking the time to play is another tool a caregiver can use to support the psyche. Play need not be elaborate or expensive. Any activity that refreshes and restores the spirit qualifies: a walk in the park, music, playing a game with your toddle, or time alone. Before making some important decisions, one of our great presidents found solace and peace of mind by going out and working in the woods. Capture the greater power of your spirit by extending it through whatever play works for you.

Remember that God's love for you is unconditional. If a patient bares your soul with questions that challenge your beliefs, it's okay. It's part of our humanness to want to have answers, but answers are not always available. Don't let this get in the way of your quest to help. Acknowledge your limits, and accept them. Every morning as I entered the big, glass double doors to the medical center, I said a little prayer to my God, asking Him to help me through the day and to guide me in being the kind of caregiver I wanted to be. Staying in touch with our spiritual side reminds us that there is a higher presence steering the universe, that we are merely instruments of this greater power, and that whatever happens is ultimately out of our hands. Understanding this also made it easy for me, as soon as the fresh air of the parking lot hit the back of my neck at the end of the day, to let everything I had experienced that day roll down my neck and off my back. "Like water off a duck's back," I used to say, and I could go home and live my personal life until the next workday. "When I works, I works hard, When I sits, I sits loose, and when I sleeps, I sleep."

Perhaps the greatest support one can muster comes from deep within the psyche, from a realm that drives us when we forget where we're going. This is the dream, the reason we are still here, the vision that appeared when we asked ourselves early on if this profession could satisfy our need to make a difference. And it's nourished by faith in ourselves and those we choose to keep around us. Remain faithful to your dream, and it will carry you through the rough spots.

We would again like to express our appreciation to my former coworker at the ICU, Nurse Practitioner Peggy, who shared her experience with a patient at another hospital. A first-year intern, who was very cocky, was managing the patient. The intern's overseeing physician had called her in as a consultant because they couldn't figure out what was wrong with the patient. The patient was in his fifties and had worked full time. He had been admitted with elevated liver enzymes. Although the intern kept insisting the problem was related to drinking, Nurse Peggy recognized the symptoms as supporting a diagnosis of hepatic congestion from very advanced congestive heart failure (CHF).

When Peggy first saw the patient, her heart sank because she knew how sick he was, something no one else had picked up. He was on death's doorstep, and it took all of Peggy's skill, persuasion, and ability to pull strings to get him transferred first to the telemetry floor and then to the CCU. After she got his insurance company to approve a transfer to Boston and pay for a heart transplant if needed, they shipped him out. The patient survived and recovered, but only after Peggy spent a week battling for his life. At the end of that week, she went home and wrote the following poignant poem.

She walked in to see the Stranger lying in the bed
So restless. So frightened. Struggling.
And the Wise one, the tired one, so skillful, knew how sick
he was

So she called the Young one, the educated one
Who didn't believe the Wise one, the tired one.

He'll be fine, said the Young one, the educated one, the
arrogant one
He's just a drinker

But the Wise one, the tired one gently stepped around the
Young one, the educated one
And the Stranger was moved to another bed, to another
place
Because someone believed how sick he was

And dawn came

And the Young one, the educated one, the arrogant one
called her
And told the Wise one, the tired one that the Stranger was
fine
But she walked in, again, another day, another room
And saw the Stranger
And saw he was gray. And saw he was cold. And saw he was
struggling
And the Wise one, the tired one, knew he was dying

She told the Young one, the educated one, the Arrogant one
that the Stranger was dying
But he didn't believe her, so Wise, so Tired, so Confident

So she moved mountains, and stepped right over the Young
one, the educated one
To move the Stranger to a new world. A strange world
Of lights. Of machines. Of noise. Of magic liquids.

Where there were more Young ones, educated ones,
Compassionate ones
Who believed her that the Stranger was dying.

And so they tried to save him.

Until another dawn came

And the Wise one, the tired one, the Confident one walked
in to see the Dying Stranger
The Not Dying Stranger
And he smiled at her weakly
I can breathe, he told her
And his eyes, and his weak heart, now healing, thanked her
And she looked at the Young one, the educated one, the
arrogant one
Now silent
Now an Observer
But she couldn't read his eyes

And she went home, still Wise, more Tired
The fireflies flickering across the rolling fields
And she walked into the garden
And began to pull weeds.

"Be glad you had the moment."
~ Steve Shagan, author

The next time you ride through Cherryfield, Maine, make an effort to locate John's farm. It's not difficult to spot, as it sits on the left atop the hill on Route 1 just after leaving the center of town. It's an imposing farm, with an extended set of buildings, including a barn and garage attached to the main structure. Clay-colored with white, ornately carved framing, black shutters, and a spectacular cupola, the buildings enclose an indoor swimming pool and overlook a meadow that looks as if it stepped out of a Heidi adventure. A bubbling brook traverses hilly fields dotted with yellow and white daisies, yellow dandelions, white Queen Anne's lace, and pink clover. Here and there one can see sheep nibbling the sweet green grass. As if it were part of the landscape, a large-scale model railroad meanders the ups and downs of the hills and valleys, even crossing a trestle at one point.

John was a stately gentleman, who carried his six-foot-two-inch frame well. At eighty-two years of age he had run into trouble with a physical condition and was in the unit in a risky attempt at repair that would subsequently spell his demise.

"What did you do for work, John?" I asked in my usual way.

"I taught at the University of Maryland," he said modestly.

"He is a PhD professor of math," his daughter, who sat in the corner of the room, proudly added. Behind her was a newspaper clipping she had posted on the bulletin board. I walked over and looked at the photograph accompanying the article. It occurred to me that the nice part about living in a small town is that when you don't know what you're doing, someone else does.

"Hey, I know this place," I quickly observed. "I pass it on the way to my property Down East. I've always admired it. Is it yours?"

John perked up. It was obviously close to his heart. "Yes, I moved there after my retirement and have made its development my hobby." He then launched into detail about how he had formed all the rails and laid every inch of track, selecting only the best metals and woods to accomplish the various functions of the model railroad. He had also carefully wired the trains to run as if they were a miniature train set, but with one important difference: one could ride on this train. The engine is a Canadian National car and pulls a box car (with room for a passenger) and an orange Long Island Caboose.

After listening to the precious details, I asked why he loved doing this, what it was about this hobby he loved so much.

"It's my psychiatrist," he simply said.

"Wow," I thought, sitting there with my mouth open. In all my years and in all my encounters with people I had met along the journey, I had never heard anything so profound, anything spoken so eloquently, put so simply. I could find no other words. "It's my psychiatrist." I realized all the preparation for my life's work, all the moments I had spent trying to earn the trust of my coworkers, my patients and their families, cleaning up messes and peeling back layers of people's lives in my attempts to help them achieve dawn, all of it had directed my energies away from myself. I had been an ordinary man in an extraordinary situation. I realized that in the process of peeling onions, one must temporarily step away or be consumed. I thought about the generations of nurses who would follow in my footsteps, and with satisfaction I knew I had made a small—yet undeniable---difference. I thought about my ocean playground to which I would soon retire and smiled in the certainty John's few words summed it all up.

Please, don't worry so much.
Because in the end,
none of us have very long on this Earth.
Life is fleeting.
And if you're ever distressed,
cast your eyes to the summer sky
when the stars are strung across the velvety night.
And when a shooting star streaks through the blackness,
turning night into day . . .
make a wish
and think of me.
Make your life
Spectacular.
I know I did.
˜ (from "Jack," written by James DeMonaco and Gary Nadeau, and recited by Robin Williams for his character's valedictory speech)

Epilogue

By the time Ray finished telling me the last story, the sun was rising, and Ray's sister, Theresa, stood and stretched, then made her way upstairs to the guest bedroom. I took their wineglasses and set them alongside mine in the sink, watching the first rays of light color the horizon and hearing the creak of springs, as Ray slid into bed. It was the dawn of a new day, a new beginning, the beginning of a new journey. Where it would take us was unknown, but what we did know for certain was that we were ready for whatever life had in store.

The End

Afterword

We would like to pay special homage to those men and women who have so selflessly cared for patients during the COVID-19 crisis. Among the usual, happy words of friends' reports inserted in holiday greeting cards two years ago were the following, and we are indebted to former critical care coworker and nurse practitioner Peg Sullivan for allowing us to close our book with them:

This has been a year unlike any other in our world. COVID has changed the world, all of us, forever. I don't usually write holiday messages in a word document, but my intent is to share this with friends, and writing it individually would be too overwhelming.

The Department of Veterans Affairs, for whom I work, has a program that began after Hurricane Katrina, called DEMPS or Disaster Emergency Medical Professionals. The program is designed to use the medical resources of the federal government and to deploy them to areas during a crisis to assist local regions. It is voluntary. I signed up years ago, and have been deployed twice before.

In early April, the call went out for medical and nursing staff to travel to NYC just as they were expecting to peak with COVID. The hospitals were overwhelmed, as was the staff, all across the city. Without knowing what role I would fill, I volunteered and was chosen, along with my nephrologist colleague and friend, Clay. We were shuttled down to NYC in early April for a 14-day deployment.

Clay and I were assigned to the Manhattan VA, a 400-bed hospital in the city, that was fully COVID. The hospital was a veterans hospital, but the patients were vets and civilians alike. Clay walked in and immediately took over a nephrology service, as one their own was out with COVID. He started a peritoneal dialysis program, as many of these critically ill patients were not only on ventilators, but were in renal failure. I was introduced to the chief of the ICUs, who, hearing my background, quickly claimed me for one of the ICUs, 11 north, a 16-bed unit. Off this unit was a 6-bed step down unit, currently closed, that became "my" unit.

Despite not working in the capacity of an ICU RN for over 30 years, I spent the next 12 days straight, from 7 am till 8 pm as an RN in this unit. I quickly formed a partnership with another DEMPS nurse from Buffalo, Jessie, who was a current ICU nurse. We quickly developed a model of care in which we each had our own patients, but we always worked as a team, and she was the "senior" nurse.

The first few minutes I walked onto the unit, I was nearly overwhelmed. The noise level was beyond description. It was loud. It was constant. It never, ever stopped. The hallway was staffed with nurses/doctors/respiratory therapists, all in heavily protective gear, face shields, caps, double masks, etc. The hall was filled to the brim with equipment, including IV machines and ventilators, which were all attached to intubated patients behind glass doors. There was a patient on a vent in the hall, waiting for a room. People were shouting up and down the hall all the time, because it was impossible to hear. This was a war zone. I knew it immediately. It was war here, and everyone was controlled, but in a chaotic way.

When Jessie and I arrived, they opened the satellite unit to accommodate more patients. We always had 4 between us. The "regular" staff nurses had up to 5 critically ill patients each. An oral surgeon was drafted to work in the ICU. A psychiatry nurse practitioner came up to work as an ICU RN, clearly out of her league but she did an exemplary job. Our unit had no running water . . . no equipment . . . no computer/telemetry monitors at the nursing station. And no drugs. We DID have PPE. Each morning we'd take a quick assessment of needs, and one of us would dash out to find some equipment. It never ended. There was no pharmacy. We needed to hand mix our own IV drugs: sedating agents, insulin, cardiac drugs, pressors.

I spent 3 ½ hours one morning mixing and hanging drugs. Sedating/paralyzing agents, pressors, insulin. All of it. We ran out of IV solution, so instead of 500-cc bags, we had only 100-cc bags, necessitating recalculations. Calculate, recheck, mix, hang and on and on.

There was a 20-minute break once each shift, to get something to eat and drink. The rest of the time we worked nonstop. These patients were the sickest I've ever seen. There was no such thing as a stable COVID patient.

And they all died, regardless of age, except for one 90-something-year-old WWII veteran, Hallsy. He made it!

And what a terrible death it was these people suffered. One minute they seemed relatively stable, and literally within 5 minutes we were coding them. At one point, there were 3 simultaneous codes going on. It was chaos. It was heartbreaking. It was *exhausting. But it was the most incredible experience I've ever had in 40 years as a nurse. The collegiality of the staff, the support they gave each other and us--- regardless of role---was nothing short of amazing.*

I tried to humanize them as best I could. One woman was a 40-year Army veteran, who had served in combat in the Persian Gulf War and had made it home alive, only to die of COVID. She was so sick, but I noticed immediately the first time I took care of her that she had manicured fingernails, a lovely lavender with sparkles. Her husband, who called and spoke with me every day to check on her (no visitors) told me she'd had them done just before contracting COVID, in preparation for a family gathering. She fought hard, but died a terrible death.

Each morning, I would walk from our hotel through the empty NYC streets to the hospital 20 minutes away. Each night I would walk back. In the hallway outside my room, I would strip off my scrubs, step into my room, grab a bag and sack them up for washing. I sprayed my shoes down out in the hall with cleanser, left them there all night. And then into the shower to clean off COVID; sterilize all my equipment; eat something and collapse.

We got tested several times on the way out, and I never (so far) contracted COVID. If I had to, I would do it all over again, not because we are heroes, but because every patient deserves care. Even those who have refused to wear a mask.

And so, Friend, that is my tale from this year. The nightmares are subsiding, but I relive it every time I see a picture on TV of an ICU or an ER.

Let's hope and pray [next year] will be a brighter year. It can't get much worse than this one has been. I plan to retire from clinical [in the spring]. I've done what I could.

Stay safe, stay healthy, wear your mask!

About the Authors (Ray and Karen Buyno): The Rest of the Story

R ay Peter Buyno grew up with eleven brothers and sisters on a farm in Illinois. He attended La Salette Seminary in Olivet, Illinois and La Salette College in Altamont, New York. For three years in the 1960s Ray was a VISTA volunteer in Appalachia and Worcester, Massachusetts, where he was immersed in all-Black neighborhoods. He was the first White man to ever live in the Black section of Hollins, Virginia and was instrumental in bringing about many needed social changes there.

Ray later worked as a taxicab driver for Town Taxi in Boston, where he met many colorful characters. He then worked as a janitor and switchboard operator for the Boston Lying-in Hospital.

In 1978 Ray received his LPN degree from Eastern Maine Vocational Technical Institute in Bangor. While preparing to get his LPN degree, Ray studied each morning from 5:00 am until 8:00 am by himself at Eastern Maine Medical Center in Bangor, as the rest of his time was used up building his house and working as a patient transporter at EMMC. In 1981 he received his RN diploma from St. Joseph Hospital's School of Nursing. His CCRN certification in critical care nursing followed in 1982, and in 2000 he received his Bachelor of Arts Degree in Nursing from the University of Maine in Orono. He was the first recipient of the Nurse of the Year Award granted by EMMC in 1989 and until 2010 served as primary relief charge nurse in the hospital's intensive care unit. He also recovered corneas for the New England Eye Bank and was an integral part of the medical center's ethics committee. Ray continues to serve as a consulting innovator for the medical center's innovation team.

Karen grew up in the Bangor area and attended the University of Maine in Orono and the University of New Brunswick in Fredericton, New Brunswick. She trained as a medical technologist at Central Maine Medical Center in Lewiston, Maine, obtaining her certification in 1975. In 1976 she was certified as a cytogenetics technologist, having trained in the state's first clinical cytogenetics laboratory at Eastern Maine Medical Center. She served as supervisor of that lab under the management of Affiliated Labs, Inc. until her retirement in 2011. She also served from 2008 until 2011 as an initiating member of the EMMC Innovation Team and as chairperson for a group of healthcare professionals interested in fostering personalized medicine in the greater Bangor area. Other books by Karen include *Even Blue Birds Sing.*

Karen met Ray through their church in 1997. During the Great Ice Storm of 1998, Ray brought wood for her woodstove and equipped her family with a kerosene heater. When he later invited her to dinner at his house, she felt secure that he was a very kind and gentle person. In retrieving something for him from his basement that evening, however, she remembers seeing little jars of body parts like esophagus, tonsil, lung, and brain, and wondered briefly if he could be a serial killer. She excused herself and left abruptly when she also found what looked like a bag of potassium chloride hanging on his refrigerator. It looked so real that Karen thought he would surely inject her with it and add her body parts to his collection.

The specimens turned out to be science fair exhibits for Ray's three children and the potassium chloride a magnet from a would-be distributor. In 2000 Ray proposed to Karen on top of Mount Washington, using a fortune cookie insert. They were married in 2004 and make their homes in South Addison, Maine and Lakeland, Florida. Between them, they have five children and---at last count---nine grandchildren.

In 2002 Karen found herself in a nursing role when she accompanied Ray to Johns Hopkins in Baltimore for major abdominal surgery. Ray was hospitalized for several days following the surgery, and he at one point ended up in the hospital's ICU with complications. Once he was released, she carefully gathered together their belongings, sat Ray in a wheelchair, and placed a potted plant (gifted to Ray from his friend JoAnn) on his lap for the trip through the airport. Ray was in pain and moved with difficulty, and she was anxious to get him home, where she could tuck him safely into his bed.

When the flight was ready to board, airline personnel allowed the pair to board first to minimize the possibility of bumping into other passengers. "Our final leg," Karen said to herself, glad the long journey would soon be over. Picking up her things, she pointed Ray at the gangplank and pushed him toward the plane. What happened next is now a series of slow-motion frames forever burned into Karen's memory. Simultaneously, she spotted the raised joint connecting one segment of the gangplank to the next, she saw Ray's mouth start to open in alarm, and she noticed the downward angle of the plank, which would ultimately set the wheelchair in a merciless acceleration. The next frame was one in which the plant flew ten feet in the air, Ray was catapulted to his knees, the chair flew against Karen's shins, and the jaws of horrified onlookers dropped. When the time warp suddenly ended, she looked up, and Ray had caught the plant! Karen cried all the way home and vowed in the future to leave caregiving to the less faint of heart.

Glossary of Nursing Vernacular

Baby Catcher----------------Obstetrician

Blood Sucker----------------Phlebotomist

Chart Dehiscence----------Patient's chart contents falling out of its folder

Cluster ----------------------A chaotic situation during which multiple things go wrong

Code Brown----------------A really big stool cleanup

Crying time-----------------Code for a painful procedure or for a major stool cleanup

Dick Doc--------------------A doc who orders a foley discontinued, followed by an order of 40 mg Lasix (a diuretic)

Eggnog----------------------Propofol: especially as used around the holidays to sedate a restless patient

FDGB------------------------Fall down go boom

Fecal Dynamics-----------The art and science of cleaning up a very messy stool and not making the situation worse. Few nurses attain this skill. (coined by Chris, CRNA)

FFH----------------------------A sweet patient's family from Hell

Frequent Flyers-------------Patients who often visit the ER with minor medical conditions

Gas Passer--------------------Anesthesiologist

Gerbil------------------------A man with a tiny manhood

Grandma's Nightmare--Creation made by an older patient who is finger painting with stool

Houdini----------------------A patient who can get out of his restraints

Noctors----------------------New ICU nurses who believe they are doctors and behave that way

Pee Wee Herman---------A doc who wears a bow tie

Prospectoscope-------------A tool for evaluating new encounters based on lessons learned (coined by Dr. Dinerman)

Powdered Sugar------------Desenex, applied to a patient's excoriated groin

SBI-------------------------------Something bad inside

Smokers & Jokers-------Patients who smoke four packs per day and constantly joke around

Super-duper------------------Nursing supervisor

Trifecta-----------------------An admission who is not only intubated, but also has central and arterial lines

U.N.-------------------------A group of physicians (notably anesthesiologists) who are from foreign countries (United Nations) and have thick accents

Vitamin V--------------------Viagra

Walkie Talkie-------------A patient in the CCU (most often), who can ambulate and who talks incessantly

Widow Maker-------------An accident in which a tree has fallen on a patient, resulting in a fatal head injury

Wish List-------------------A list of things a night nurse wants the attending doc to consider the following morning

Bibliography

[1]Nietzsche, Friedrich, BrainyQuote.com, Xplore Inc, 2015. http://www.brainyquote.com/quotes/quotes/f/friedrichn103819.ht ml, accessed December 16, 2015.

[2]Benner, Patricia, *From Novice to Expert*, Menlo Park, California, Addison-Wesley, 1984.

[3]Pettigrew, Jan, PhD, RN, "Coming Alongside in Suffering: The Power of the Nurse's Presence," Las Vegas, Nevada, April 13--16, 1998, The National Professional Education Institute and the National Critical Care Institute of Education presents the 24th annual Critical Care Update Conference.

[4]Pettigrew, Jan, PhD, RN, personal communication, September 2022.

[5]Muggeridge, Malcolm, "Something Beautiful for God." https://www.christianitytoday.com/history/issues/issue-65/ministries-of-mercy-mother-teresa.html.

[6]Pettigrew, Jan, PhD, RN, "Intensive Nursing Care: The Ministry of Presence," *Critical Care Nursing Clinics of North America*, Vol. 2, No. 3, September 1990.

[7]Suzuki, Shunryu, *Zen Mind, Beginner's Mind: Informal Talks on Zen Meditation and Practice*, Shambhala, June 28, 2011.

[8]Pettigrew, Jan, PhD, RN, personal communication, December 2022.

[9]O'Leary, Rand, FACHE, Senior Vice President, Northern Light Health, and President, Northern Light Eastern Maine Medical Center, "Currents," October 3--9, 2022.

[10]Frankl, Viktor E., *Man's Search for Meaning: An Introduction to Logotherapy* (a newly revised edition of *From Death Camp to Existentialism*), Simon and Shuster, Inc., New York, New York, 1984.

[11]O'Connor, Nancy, (*Letting Go with Love: The Grieving Process*), La Mariposa Press, Tucson, Arizona, 1994.

[12]Pettigrew, JM: A Phenomenological Study of the Nurse's Presence with Persons Experiencing Suffering [unpublished doctoral dissertation], Denton, TX, Texas Woman's University College of Nursing, 1988.

[13]Copies of *Passing Showers* may be obtained by writing to Daryl at dewitmer@aol.com.

[14]C. G. Jung, *Psychology and Religion: West and East*, Princeton University Press, 2014, page 339.

[15]Cardillo, Donna, RN, *A Daybook for Beginning Nurses*, ISBN 978-1-930538-87-0. Copyright 2010 Sigma Theta Tau International, page 30.

[16]http://www.trueghosttales.com/paranormal/vanishing-into-the-4th-dimension/.

[17]Koontz, Dean, "The Frankenstein Series 5-Book Bundle: Frankenstein: Prodigal Son, City of Night, Dead and Alive, Lost Souls, The Dead Town," p. 649, Bantam, 2012, https://www.azquotes.com/quote/391451.

[18]Lepre, George, *Fragging: Why U.S. Soldiers Assaulted Their Officers in Vietnam*, Lubbock, Texas Tech University Press, 2011.

Other Treasures

"A friend is one who overlooks your broken fence and admires the flowers in your garden."
~Author unknown

Before I became a nurse, I worked for Steven's Studio, Maine's premier photography studio for senior portraits in high schools and colleges. The person who trained me said, "There is something beautiful in everyone. You just have to capture that in your portraits." I never forgot that concept and carried it with me into my nursing career. To be honest, I never met a nurse I didn't like.

The following sentiments were delivered to me at my retirement celebration in two bound books. The signers saw something in me---despite thirty-eight years of faults and shortcomings---that they could celebrate and honor. But these thoughts say more about the people who penned them than they do about me. It is because of all of them that this book exists, for I took the best of them and molded it into my personhood. I took the best parts of their actions, spirits, and words. Until I saw what they did and how they made others feel, I never knew what to emulate. It is with a humble heart that I am grateful for their example. I share their words now to show that presencing in small ways with coworkers can sometimes make a huge difference. Thank you.

Thank you so much for taking care of the people who are taking care of the people. Just know that you are so amazing at your job, always in a calm manner.
~Beth Fuller, RN, ICU

I worked with you for 18 years in the ICU. I babysat your kids when I was in high school.
~April Stanhope, Secretary, ICU

Your sense of humor and calmness in times of crisis helped me a great deal when I started as a brand-new attending. You sent me a very funny, thoughtful note on "Doctor's Day." That meant a lot.
~Sigrid Noack, MD, ICU Intensivist

I remember being a teenager and seeing you ride your bike with your kids in Exeter, Maine. I thought, "That guy is a cool ICU nurse. I hope to be like him someday." Love, the farmer from Exeter . . .
~Karyn Chadbourne, RN, ICU

The end of an era. I have known you my whole life as a nurse. No one shares the same memories with me that you do. Been through a bunch of bosses and trained some manager "Baboons." As Mary Ellen (ICU Dept. Manager) said to me, "You always think Ray can't do anything wrong." You were a great classmate, coworker and friend. I will never forget the baby shower for my son Ethan. I remember the Valentine's Day dances with my daughter Katy and you including my father. Playing Santa with the kids. Love,
~Pam Wallace, RN, Charge Nurse, ICU days (Ray's boss)

It's been a pleasure getting to know you and for you finally getting my name right after 10 years.
~Sheila Clapp, RN, ICU nights

You have been a charm to work with. Make sure you poop every day or I will come to make you happy. You will be missed more than you know.
~ ("Pea Brain") Darleen McGarrigle, RN, ICU

WOW--what a wonderful career you had at EMMC! So many accomplishments.
~Debbie Johnson, President and CEO, EMMC

Thanks for all the great assignments.
~Martin Keresey, RN, ICU

You have been the most considerate charge nurse to follow. Always sharpening my pencils for me and having everything tidy and ready to go.
~Angela Harding, RN, Relief Charge Nurse, ICU nights

It's been a pleasure having known you and having you in my life. Love you,
~Sandy Rothera, Esq., RN

A quality control guy in ICU.
~Joe from Monroe (Isgro), Respiratory Therapist, ICU

You were a great mentor---quiet and strong, patient and considerate.
~Sandy Benton, MSN, RN, Lifeflight

You have always been the go-to guy. Nobody can fill your shoes.
~Tricia Bubar, RN, ICU

You are a nursing "officer and a gentleman" even though you gave a better evaluation for my wife (Dr. Savitha) than me.
~Thomas Rajan, MD

Thanks for sticking by me and helping me through some rough patient cases.
~Michelle Lizotte, RN, ICU

I have known you for 25 years. You ran the unit in your own style.
~Cynthia Rice, Unit Secretary, ICU

This place will fall apart without you.
~Jen Lee, RN, ICU nights

We have been through so much: births, deaths, tragedies and joys. Few colleagues have had such a lasting impact.
~Debbie Leighton, RN, ICU

CONTRARY to what everybody says, you were <u>always</u> great to work with. Please accept best wishes from my fellow "vulture," Laura.
~John Macone, RN, New England Organ Bank

You are such an important part of making me the nurse I am today. I have certainly come a long way, and yet you seem no different. You are the rock this unit has been built on. This is to you and your monkey.
~Dawn Brown, RN, ICU

How can someone begin to thank you for everything you have done?
~Jackie Pushard, RN, Clinical Supervisor, ICU

We'll miss you and that Barry White voice. We love you.
~Lisa Saunders, RN, ICU

You were always able to help. Your common sense and insights.
~Leon Binette, RN, ICU

TOO many memories on evenings.
~Cathy Brooks, RN, ICU

It has been a pleasure working with you.
~Jennifer Fogel, RN, Nursing Administration

Thank you for all you have taught me.
~Amy Cangelosi, RN, PICU

Enjoy sleeping in every morning.
~Kathy Killarney, RN, ICU

First knew you at Boston Lying-in Hospital in Boston when you were evening switchboard operator.
~Sue Wilson, RN, Rosen NICU (1978-2010)

I will take all that I have learned from you and apply it to my own practice.
~Heather Haskins, RN, ICU

YOU are totally the MFIC.
~ ("Animal") Anna Moses, RN, ICU

DON'T get your days mixed up.
~Carol Silsby, RN, ICU

You're a leader in every aspect. An example for the rest of us, just in who you are.
~Sandi Carver, CRNA

Mondays and Tuesdays will always be Ray days for me. My transition to ICU was made so easy due to your education, cool demeanor and sense of humor.
~Lois Latour, Social Worker, ICU

It has always been fun working with you and sharing information.
~Michael Moreau, PAC, ICU

Thank you for all you have done for me, smoothing out the rough spots and most importantly maintaining a positive attitude through all the ups and downs of critical care.
~Tom Frey, MD

You are the glue that kept ICU together. The man to go to with equipment questions, words of wisdom and ICU pearls.
~Carole West (Starno), RN, ICU

We will miss your strengths and talents around here.
~David Lee, RN, ICU nights

Eat pie every day. You are a gentleman and a nurse who I respect and have learned a lot from.
~Lisa Oliver, RN, ICU nights

You will be 100 times busier.
~Deb Sanford, RN, Director of Nursing, EMMC

You have big shoes to fill.
~Helen Black, Unit Secretary, ICU

You are the man and no one will replace you or your flannel-lined jammie scrubs.
~ ("Canadian RN from Sas-katchew-wan") Alyson Cameron, RN, ICU

I do believe you are one of my favorite charge nurses. How dare you leave me just when I was getting comfortable? You have been good to me.
~Karen Boudreau, RN, ICU

Whenever I asked you for help, you never said no. Your Addison Girl,
~Jen Murphy, RN, ICU

One thing I missed since moving to human resources has been our long talks. You are one of my oldest and dearest friends.
~Kim Kneeland, Unit Secretary, ICU

I will value and use your words of wisdom.
~Tammy Doughty, RN, ICU

We will miss you not only for your medical care of patients but also because of your spirituality.
~Robert Bach, MD

EMMC will not be the same without you
~Brenda Homsted, RN

You grab ahold of new technology like a kid grabs a new puppy, and you get the same enjoyment.
~ ("Trooper") Lori Strout, RN, ICU

Oh, Ray, you are such a legend.
~Cameron Dalton (Clough), RN, ICU nights

I have to say you taught me so much about being an ICU nurse.
~Tiffany Cyr, RN, ICU

The staff knew they could count on you, and that is a quality you were known for.
~Wendy Arno, RN, ICU

You are the only one that kept everyone else from going crazy.
~Tammi Pearson, Unit Secretary, ICU

Brother Ray, you will be thought of every time I pull into "our parking spot."
~Paul Finden, RN, CCU

Thank you so much for the great advice and tips on becoming a better nurse and person. We have had many laughs and "girly" talks.
~Maggie Smith-Watkins, RN, ICU

Will miss you a lot.
~Zita Williams, RN, ICU

You have always been a wealth of knowledge when it comes to the ins and outs of ICU.
~Hanna McLaughlin, RN, ICU

In my 40 years of clinical experience, I offer this. The good air goes in, the bad air goes out and the blood goes round and round. Good Luck.
~Eddie Harrow, MD

I have always enjoyed you a lot, your sense of humor and attention to detail! You are a class act and one of a kind.
~Paula Rouleau, RN, Charge Nurse, ICU nights

Thanks for all that you have done to keep the ICU the exceptional place that it is. Your shoes will be impossible to fill. Love,
~Kathleen Stewart, Secretary, ICU nights

Don't want to see you on the other side of the fence. Nice working with you.
~Deb (Joy) Smith, Unit Secretary/Monitor Tech, Grant 4 cardiac

I will miss you very much. Maybe see you in the curtain shop.
~Cindy L, Housekeeper, Grant 8 pediatrics

I will think of you often. Where have the years gone?
~Deb Chase, RN, Case Manager, ICU

You have been an inspiration. I thoroughly enjoyed working with you.
~Jaime Hanson, RN, CCU

You are like a fixture in the ICU. You were my go-to person when I needed something done.
~ ("Jimmy") Sue Williams, RN, Department Manager, ICU

I enjoyed working with you over the years on the unit and in our ethics program. You were a faithful member.
~Rev. Rex Garrett, Chaplain, EMMC

You were a steady guiding force when I first came to EMMC.
~Mari-Ann Faloon, RN, CCU

You always believed in me and I appreciate your soft-spoken approach.
~Kim Doughty, RN, ICU

Your kind and gentle spirit has been a beacon of hope for me and many others during a bad day in ICU. Much Love,
~Sue Mishio, RN, ICU

Your goal to always make the life of the bedside nurse a bit easier will never be underestimated.
~Crystal Landry, RN, CEO, Lincoln Maine Hospital

Thanks for being the go-to guy in ICU.
~Dee Webber, RN, CCU

Thanks for sharing the journey and for always protecting your nurses.
~Lynne Estes, RN, ICU

I've enjoyed working with you. Thanks for the tea and food.
~Rob Hand, MD

It's hard to believe you are retiring. What an accomplishment!
~Helen Qualey McKinnon, RN, Nursing Administration

A steady force in the ICU.
~Carol Jordan, RN, ICU and Lifeflight

Thanks for all your help. You made such a difference. Love,
~ ("Holy Holly") Holly Mills, RN, ICU

You made it fun to come to work.
~Rena Dubay, RN, ICU

There is not a day that goes by that I don't hear someone say, "I miss Ray."
~Elaine O'Connell, RN, ICU

You are one of a kind. A wonderful caring person.
~Andrea Longley, RN, ICU

Thanks for making it a fun place to work. Your smile and laughter will be greatly missed.
~Paige Dunn, RN, ICU

You never faltered and always excelled. Love you,
~Sue Dunning, RN, ICU

When I came around the corner from the locker room at the beginning of my day, I knew you would always be the same person.
~Valerie Klick, RN, ICU

You like to play with us all the time.
~Debbie, RN, ICU

Your energy and sense of humor made coming to work fun & enjoyable.
~ ("Little Dicker") Jen Dicker, RN, ICU

Can you give me a nickname?
~Julie S., RN, ICU

Your knowledge and stories have been beneficial and definitely entertaining.
~Erica Parker, RN, ICU

Thanks for all you taught me.
~Jay Fonseca, RN, ICU

You are a wonderful charge nurse.
~Michelle (Rioux) Dunning, RN, ICU

It's been a great pleasure working with you. I hope you continue to be "bis-y."
~ ("Super G") Alan Garber, MD

Thanks for all the mentoring and the smiles.
~Dawn Ravan, RN, ICU

Thanks for all the memories. I certainly could not have done everything that I did without your and the other nurses' help.
~Dr. Furtick

Will miss the fun times.
~Tyra, Housekeeper, CCU/CSU

Happy trails.
~Theresa Clark, RN, ICU

I really appreciate all the teaching and advice at times.
~Jay Hughes, RN, ICU

RAY-licious. You have always been my biggest cheerleader. Thank you for all your advice and support. I wish I had a dad like you. Love,
~Brooke Michaud (Rankin), RN, ICU

We will miss you a lot.
~Zita Prescott, RN, ICU

You have always been a pleasure to work with.
~Kelly Hargrove, RN, ICU

You have made a great impact.
~Lorraine Rodgerson, RN, former Director of Nursing, EMMC

Thank you for all your assistance.
~Judy Shaw, RN, ICU

You have made the intolerable days tolerable.
~Danny Edwards, RN, ICU

Stay healthy and enjoy each day.
~Pam Vickers, RN, ICU

What will ICU do without you?
~Kathy Pushor, RN, CCU

You are so sweet and kind. Thank you for those times that have affected me in ways that I think and hope have improved me as a person. I miss our "bantering" . . . which I did mostly to try to get you going.
~Marie Ewing, RN, ICU

I still don't see how you can do it if I can't.
~Steve Dunning, RN, CCU

You have made me feel welcomed in ICU.
~Rena Dubay, RN, ICU

It has been a joy working with you.
~Debbie Clegg, Unit Secretary, ICU

Wishing you the best of everything you've given to all your patients.
~Eloise Griffin, RN, CCU

It has been a pleasure to work with you.
~Deb Flint, Respiratory Therapist, ICU

Enjoy your retirement.
~Autumn Lake, RN, ICU

All the best in your retirement.
~James Sears, MD

You have been a vital force in this unit.
~Kerry Mavor, RN, ICU

I hope you enjoy your memories of your extended stay in ICU.
~Dianna Vassar, RN, ICU

First and foremost, go wipe your nose. Secondly, you suck. Thirdly I'm going to miss you. Please don't leave me here with Pam.
~Lisa Buzzell, RN, ICU

It has been a pleasure working with you all these years. You always made me feel like I was part of your team.
~Deanna Bean, Housekeeper, ICU

I consider it a pleasure working with you and teasing you. Check under your bed to see if I left anything under your bed last night.
~Margie Roberts, RN, CCU

I have never seen you tense, upset or any other mood except being professional and jolly.
~Reddy Yeruva, MD

You are one of a kind. I will miss you, especially the deadpan sense of quiet humor, the energy and often uplifting wit.
~Ruth Talley, MD

Thanks for being such a great mentor. Love,
~Sarah Cummings, RN, ICU

You will be missed.
~Randee Jensen, RN, ICU nights

You will be missed.
~Alexei Bogolioubov, MD

It has been a pleasure working with you over the years.
~Delight Joslyn, RN

Incontinence care will never be the same.
~Ken Grunder, RN, CCU

You will be greatly missed.
~Carmen Morgan, RN, ICU

You will be missed in many ways by many people.
~Delaine Follero, RN, ICU nights

You will be missed greatly. You are an inspiration to all nurses. I only hope that someday I can be half as good of a nurse that you are.
~ ("Alice") Elissa Spofford McCall, RN, ICU

You should be proud, and also EMMC. Your dedication has shown.
~Gretchen Dyer-Gagnon, RN, CCU

When I first worked in ICU, you asked me if I baked pies. Then you told me we were having "potluck" on Saturday and would I bring in a pie? I agreed. Later I found out that the "potluck" was a spur of the moment idea . . . Ray went around telling others Barbara was bringing in a pie so why don't you all bring in something and we could have potluck. Isn't this classic Ray?
~Barbara Joyce, RN, ICU

Author photos courtesy of Samantha Mahar

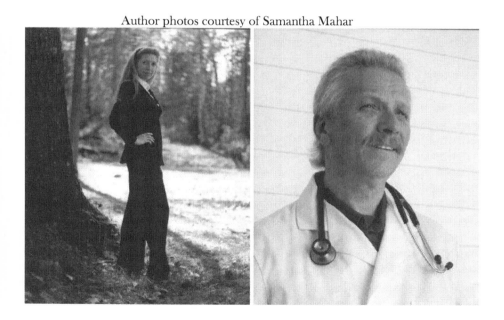

Made in the USA
Middletown, DE
26 September 2023

39404062R00196